THE GERD DIET COOKBOOK FOR BEGINNERS

A Complete Guide For Managing Acid Reflux And Enjoy Delicious Gut-Friendly Meals

Derek Klein

TABLE OF CONTENTS

Introduction

Welcome to The GERD Diet Cookbook For Beginners, your comprehensive guide to managing Gastroesophageal Reflux Disease (GERD) through delicious and nutritious meals. If you're one of the millions of people suffering from acid reflux, heartburn, and discomfort, this cookbook is designed to help you take control of your diet and alleviate your symptoms.

GERD affects millions of people worldwide, causing discomfort, pain, and anxiety. While medication and lifestyle changes are often necessary, diet plays a crucial role in managing symptoms and preventing flare-ups. Unfortunately, many people with GERD find it challenging to navigate the complex landscape of trigger foods, dietary restrictions, and confusing nutrition advice.

That's why we created The GERD Diet Cookbook. Our goal is to provide you with a practical, easy-to-follow guide to managing GERD through diet. Inside these pages, you'll discover:

- Over 50 delicious, GERD-friendly recipes carefully crafted to soothe your stomach and reduce inflammation
- A comprehensive guide to identifying and avoiding trigger foods
- Tips for balancing your diet with nutrient-rich, easy-to-digest foods

- Strategies for managing symptoms and improving your quality of life
- Expert advice from healthcare professionals and registered dietitians

Our recipes are designed to be easy to prepare, flavorful, and nutritious, using ingredients that are readily available in most supermarkets. We've also included meal planning tips, grocery shopping guides, and cooking techniques to make your culinary journey as smooth as possible.

By following the principles and recipes in this cookbook, you'll be empowered to take control of your diet, alleviate your symptoms, and enjoy a healthier, more comfortable life. So let's get started on this culinary journey together

What Is GERD?

Gastroesophageal Reflux Disease (GERD) is a chronic and often debilitating condition that affects millions of people worldwide. It occurs when the ring of muscle that separates the esophagus and stomach, called the lower esophageal sphincter (LES), fails to function properly, allowing stomach acid to flow back up into the esophagus.

This backflow of acid can cause a range of uncomfortable and painful symptoms, including heartburn, chest pain, difficulty swallowing, and regurgitation of food. If left untreated, GERD can lead to serious complications, such as esophagitis, stricture, and Barrett's esophagus, a precursor to esophageal cancer.

GERD is often associated with lifestyle factors, such as diet, obesity, and stress, and can be managed through a combination of dietary changes, lifestyle modifications, and medical treatment. In this book, we will explore the ins and outs of GERD, its causes, symptoms, and management strategies, with a special focus on the role of diet in preventing and alleviating this condition.

By understanding what GERD is and how it affects the body, we can take the first step towards managing this condition and regaining control over our health and wellbeing.

Symptoms And Complications

Symptoms of GERD:
- Heartburn: a burning sensation in the chest and throat that occurs when stomach acid flows back up into the esophagus
- Regurgitation: the sensation of food or acid backing up into the mouth or throat
- Difficulty Swallowing: trouble swallowing food or liquids, especially if they are hot or spicy
- Chest Pain: pain or discomfort in the chest or arms that can be mistaken for a heart attack

- Coughing or Wheezing: coughing or wheezing can occur when stomach acid flows into the lungs
- Hoarseness: a raspy or strained voice
- Sour Taste: a sour or bitter taste in the mouth
- Burping: frequent burping or belching

Complications of GERD:
- Esophagitis: inflammation of the esophagus that can lead to scarring and narrowing
- Stricture: a narrowing of the esophagus that can make swallowing difficult
- Barrett's Esophagus: a precancerous condition where the lining of the esophagus changes to resemble the lining of the intestines
- Esophageal Cancer: cancer that develops in the esophagus
- Asthma: GERD can trigger or exacerbate asthma symptoms
- Chronic Cough: a persistent cough can develop in some people with GERD
- Sleep Disturbances: GERD can disrupt sleep patterns and reduce quality of life
- Tooth Decay: stomach acid can erode tooth enamel and lead to tooth decay
- Vocal Cord Damage: stomach acid can damage the vocal cords and lead to hoarseness or a raspy voice.

It's important to note that some people with GERD may not experience any symptoms at all, or they may only experience mild symptoms. In severe cases, GERD can lead to serious complications that can impact quality of life and overall health. If you're experiencing any of these symptoms, it's important to talk to your doctor about getting a proper diagnosis and treatment plan.

Chapter One

Understanding GERD Diet

Gastroesophageal Reflux Disease (GERD) is a chronic condition characterized by the backflow of stomach acid into the esophagus, leading to symptoms like heartburn, chest pain, and difficulty swallowing. While medication and lifestyle changes are essential for managing GERD, diet plays a crucial role in alleviating symptoms and preventing complications.

Key Principles of GERD Diet:
1. Avoid Trigger Foods: Identify and avoid foods that trigger GERD symptoms, such as citrus fruits, tomatoes, chocolate, caffeine, alcohol, and spicy or fatty foods.
2. Choose Acid-Reducing Foods: Include foods that reduce acid production and alleviate symptoms, like ginger, aloe vera juice, licorice root, and fatty fish.
3. Increase Fiber Intake: Fiber-rich foods like fruits, vegetables, legumes, and whole grains improve digestion and reduce symptoms.
4. Incorporate Probiotics: Probiotic-rich foods like yogurt, kefir, sauerkraut, and kimchi promote gut health and alleviate symptoms.
5. Stay Hydrated: Drink plenty of water and other fluids to dilute stomach acid and aid digestion.

6. Eat Small, Frequent Meals: Divide daily food intake into smaller, more frequent meals to reduce symptoms.
7. Maintain a Healthy Weight: Excess weight can exacerbate GERD symptoms; aim for a healthy BMI through a balanced diet and regular exercise.

Foods To Eat

- Lean proteins (poultry, fish, beans)
- Whole grains (brown rice, quinoa, whole wheat)
- Vegetables (leafy greens, broccoli, carrots)
- Fruits (bananas, melons, berries)
- Low-fat dairy (yogurt, kefir, milk)
- Healthy fats (avocado, nuts, olive oil)

Foods To Avoid

- Citrus fruits and juices
- Tomatoes and tomato-based products
- Fried and fatty foods
- Chocolate
- Caffeine
- Alcohol
- Spicy and acidic foods

Meal Planning And Snacking

- Plan meals in advance to avoid trigger foods

- Choose snacks that are low in acid and fat, like fruits, nuts, and veggies
- Avoid eating close to bedtime

By following these guidelines and working with a healthcare provider or registered dietitian, individuals with GERD can develop a personalized diet plan that alleviates symptoms, promotes healing, and improves overall quality of life.

Importance Of Diet In Managing GERD

Diet plays a crucial role in managing Gastroesophageal Reflux Disease (GERD). A well-planned diet can help alleviate symptoms, prevent complications, and improve overall quality of life. Here are some key aspects of diet's importance in managing GERD:

1. **Trigger Foods:** Identify and avoid foods that trigger GERD symptoms, such as:
    - Citrus fruits and juices
    - Tomatoes and tomato-based products
    - Fried and fatty foods
    - Chocolate
    - Caffeine
    - Alcohol
    - Spicy and acidic foods
2. **Acid-Reducing Foods:** Include foods that reduce acid production and alleviate symptoms:

- Ginger
- Aloe vera juice
- Licorice root
- Fatty fish (like salmon and mackerel)
- Oatmeal
- Whole grains

3. **Fiber-Rich Foods:** Increase fiber intake to improve digestion and reduce symptoms:
    - Fruits (like bananas, melons, and berries)
    - Vegetables (like broccoli, carrots, and sweet potatoes)
    - Legumes (like beans, lentils, and peas)
    - Whole grains (like brown rice, quinoa, and whole wheat)

4. **Probiotics:** Incorporate probiotic-rich foods to promote gut health:
    - Yogurt
    - Kefir
    - Sauerkraut
    - Kimchi
    - Kombucha

5. **Hydration:** Drink plenty of water and other fluids to dilute stomach acid and aid digestion:
    - Aim for at least 8-10 glasses of water per day
    - Herbal teas and low-acidity juices (like almond milk and coconut water) can also be helpful

6. **Meal Timing and Size:** Eat smaller, more frequent meals to reduce symptoms:
    - Avoid heavy meals close to bedtime
    - Eat 3-4 main meals and 2-3 snacks per day

7. **Weight Management:** Maintain a healthy weight to reduce pressure on the lower esophageal sphincter:
   - Aim for a BMI between 18.5 and 24.9
   - Consult a healthcare professional for personalized guidance

By incorporating these dietary changes, individuals with GERD can experience significant symptom relief and improved quality of life. It's essential to work with a healthcare provider or a registered dietitian to develop a personalized diet plan that addresses specific needs and health goals.

A balanced GERD diet offers numerous benefits, including:

1. **Reduced symptoms:** Alleviates heartburn, acid reflux, and discomfort.
2. **Improved digestion:** Enhances nutrient absorption and regular bowel movements.
3. **Inflammation reduction:** Decreases inflammation in the esophagus and stomach lining.
4. **Weight management:** Supports healthy weight loss and maintenance.
5. **Improved overall health:** Reduces the risk of chronic diseases like diabetes, heart disease, and certain cancers.
6. **Enhanced mental well-being:** Decreases stress, anxiety, and depression related to GERD symptoms.
7. **Better sleep:** Promotes restful sleep and improves sleep quality.

8. **Increased energy:** Provides essential nutrients for optimal energy levels.

9. **Improved medication effectiveness:** Enhances the efficacy of GERD medications.

10. **Long-term symptom management:** Helps manage symptoms over time, reducing the risk of complications.

11. **Improved quality of life:** Enhances overall well-being, allowing individuals to enjoy daily activities with reduced discomfort.

Chapter Two

Delicious Breakfast Recipes

1. Oatmeal With Banana And Honey

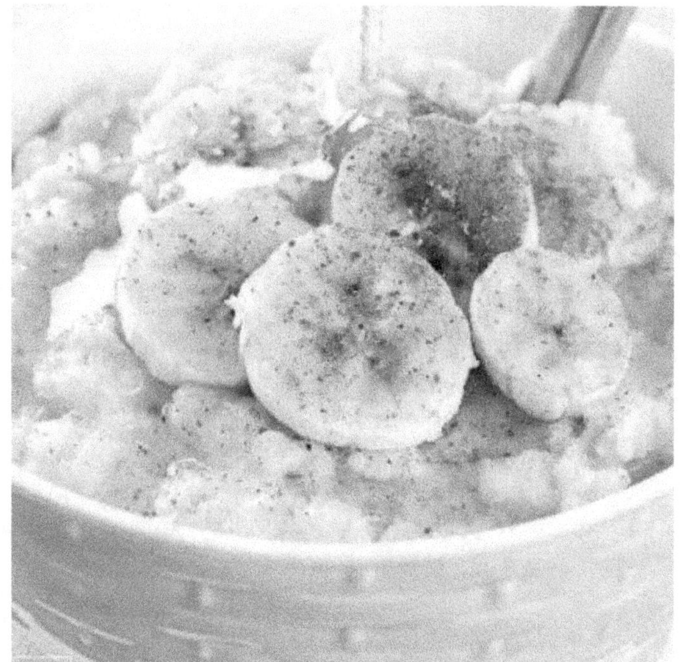

Ingredients:
- 1 cup rolled oats
- 1 cup low-fat milk (or water)

- 1 ripe banana, sliced
- 1-2 tablespoons honey
- Pinch of salt

Instructions:
1. In a pot, bring the milk (or water) to a simmer over medium heat.
2. Add the oats and salt. Stir to combine.
3. Reduce heat to low and cook, stirring occasionally, until the oats have absorbed most of the liquid and have a creamy consistency (about 5-7 minutes).
4. Add the sliced banana and stir to combine.
5. Cook for an additional 1-2 minutes, until the banana is heated through.
6. Stir in the honey until dissolved.
7. Serve hot and enjoy.

Tips:
- Use a non-stick pot to prevent the oats from sticking and to make cleanup easier.
- Adjust the amount of milk or water to achieve your desired consistency.
- Add other toppings like chopped nuts or seeds for added crunch and nutrition.

2. Whole Grain Toast With Avocado And Scrambled Eggs

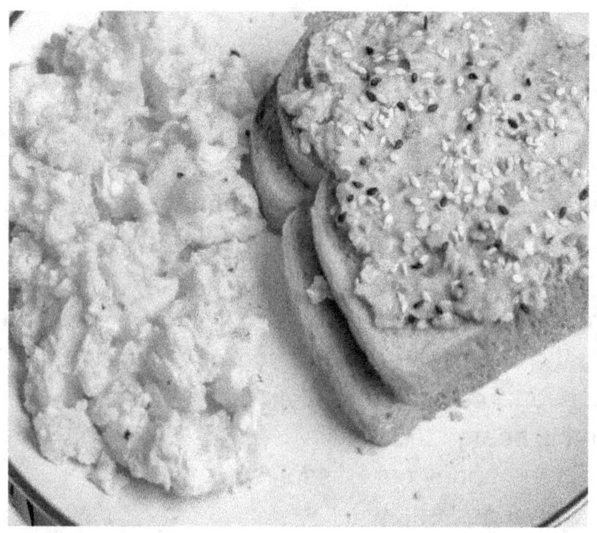

Ingredients:
- 2 slices whole grain bread (low-acidity, low-fat)
- 1 ripe avocado, mashed
- 2 eggs
- 1 tablespoon low-fat butter or non-stick cooking spray
- Salt and pepper to taste

Instructions:
1. Toast the bread until lightly browned.
2. Spread the mashed avocado on top of the toast.
3. In a bowl, whisk the eggs and season with salt and pepper.
4. Add the low-fat butter or non-stick cooking spray to a non-stick pan over medium heat.

5. Pour in the eggs and scramble until cooked through.
6. Place the scrambled eggs on top of the avocado toast.
7. Serve and enjoy!

Tips:
- Choose whole grain bread that is low in acidity and fat.
- Use ripe avocados to avoid any acidity.
- Cook scrambled eggs with low-fat milk or water to avoid adding extra fat.
- Eat slowly and mindfully to help alleviate GERD symptoms.

3. Greek Yogurt With Berries And Granola

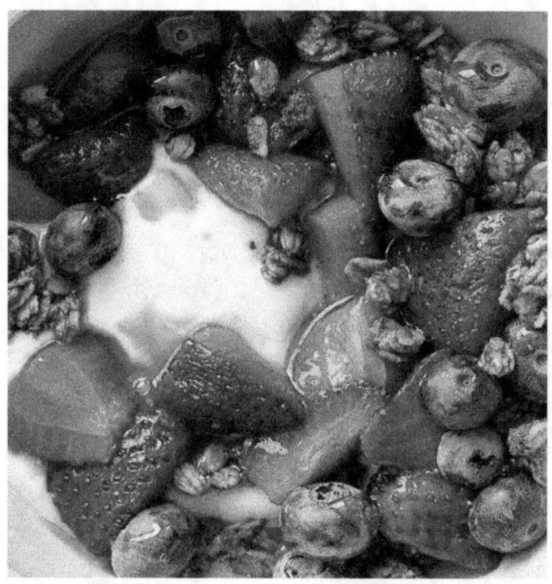

Ingredients:
- 1 cup Greek yogurt (low-fat, low-acidity)
- 1 cup mixed berries (low-acidity, such as blueberries, strawberries, raspberries)
- 2 tablespoons granola (low-fat, low-acidity)
- 1 tablespoon honey (optional)

Instructions:
1. In a bowl, mix together the Greek yogurt and honey (if using).
2. Top with mixed berries.
3. Sprinkle granola over the berries.
4. Serve and enjoy!

Tips:
- Choose a low-fat, low-acidity Greek yogurt to avoid triggering GERD symptoms.
- Select low-acidity berries, such as blueberries, strawberries, and raspberries.
- Opt for a low-fat, low-acidity granola to avoid adding extra fat and acidity.
This recipe is a delicious and soothing breakfast or snack option that should help alleviate GERD symptoms. The Greek yogurt provides a calming effect on the esophagus and stomach, while the berries offer a sweet and tangy flavor without triggering acidity. The granola adds a satisfying crunch without adding extra fat or acidity.

4. Smoothie Bowl With Almond Milk, Spinach, And Almond Butter Topping

Ingredients:
- 1 cup almond milk (low-acidity, low-fat)
- 1 cup fresh spinach leaves (low-acidity, easy to digest)
- 1/2 banana, sliced (low-acidity, easy to digest)
- 1 tablespoon almond butter (low-acidity, healthy fat)
- 1/2 cup sliced almonds (low-acidity, crunchy topping)
- 1 tablespoon chia seeds (low-acidity, fiber-rich)

Instructions:
1. In a blender, combine almond milk, spinach, and banana. Blend until smooth.
2. Pour the smoothie into a bowl.
3. Top with almond butter, sliced almonds, and chia seeds.
4. Serve and enjoy!

Tips:
- Use almond milk instead of regular milk to avoid triggering GERD symptoms.
- Add spinach for its calming effects on the esophagus and stomach.
- Choose a ripe banana for easy digestion.
- Opt for almond butter as a healthy fat source that's low in acidity.
- Add sliced almonds and chia seeds for crunch and fiber without triggering acidity.

This smoothie bowl is a nutritious and filling breakfast or snack option that should help alleviate GERD symptoms. The almond milk and spinach provide a soothing effect, while the banana and almond butter offer natural sweetness and healthy fats. The sliced almonds and chia seeds add crunch and fiber without triggering acidity.

5. Whole Grain Cereal With Low-Fat Milk And Sliced Banana

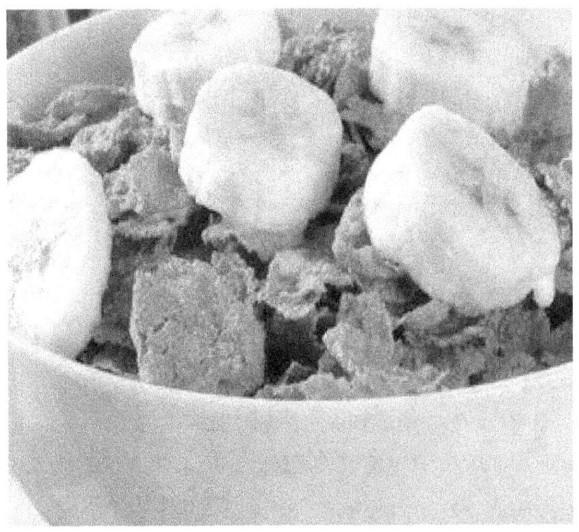

Ingredients:
- 1 cup whole grain cereal (low-acidity, high-fiber)
- 1 cup low-fat milk (1% or 2% milk fat)
- 1 ripe banana, sliced
- Optional: 1 tablespoon honey or maple syrup
(low-acidity sweeteners)

Instructions:
1. Pour the low-fat milk into a bowl.
2. Add the whole grain cereal and stir to combine.
3. Top with sliced banana.
4. If desired, add a drizzle of honey or maple syrup.
5. Serve and enjoy!

Tips:

- Choose a whole grain cereal that is low in acidity and high in fiber.
- Select a low-fat milk to avoid triggering GERD symptoms.
- Use a ripe banana for easy digestion.
- Opt for honey or maple syrup as low-acidity sweeteners, if desired.
- Eat slowly and mindfully to help alleviate GERD symptoms.

This recipe is a quick and easy breakfast option that should help alleviate GERD symptoms. The whole grain cereal provides fiber and a soothing effect, while the low-fat milk and banana offer a creamy and easy-to-digest base. The optional honey or maple syrup add a touch of sweetness without triggering acidity.

6. Grilled Chicken Breast With Roasted Vegetables And Quinoa

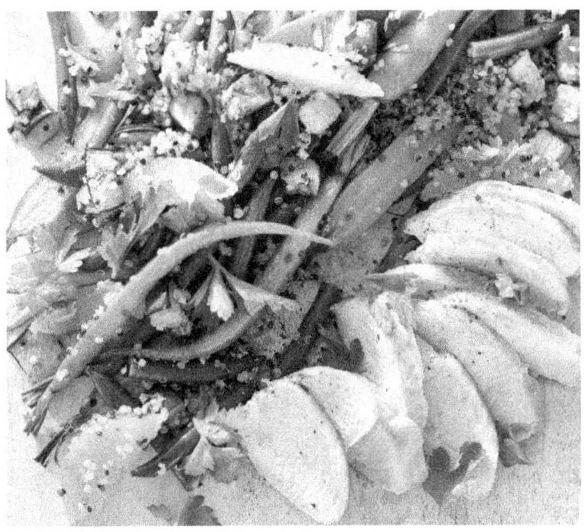

Ingredients:
- 4 boneless, skinless chicken breasts (low-fat, easy to digest)
- 2 cups mixed vegetables (low-acidity, such as bell peppers, zucchini, carrots)
- 1 cup quinoa (low-acidity, high-fiber)
- 2 tablespoons olive oil (low-acidity, healthy fat)
- Salt and pepper to taste

Instructions:
1. Preheat the grill to medium-high heat.
2. Season chicken breasts with salt and pepper.
3. Grill chicken for 5-6 minutes per side, or until cooked through.

4. Toss vegetables in olive oil and roast in the oven at 400°F (200°C) for 20-25 minutes, or until tender.
5. Cook quinoa according to package instructions.
6. Serve grilled chicken with roasted vegetables and quinoa.

Tips:
- Choose lean protein sources like chicken breast to avoid triggering GERD symptoms.
- Select low-acidity vegetables like bell peppers, zucchini, and carrots.
- Cook quinoa according to package instructions to ensure it's easy to digest.
- Use olive oil as a healthy fat source that's low in acidity.
- Eat slowly and mindfully to help alleviate GERD symptoms.

7. Whole Grain Waffles With Fresh Berries And Yogurt

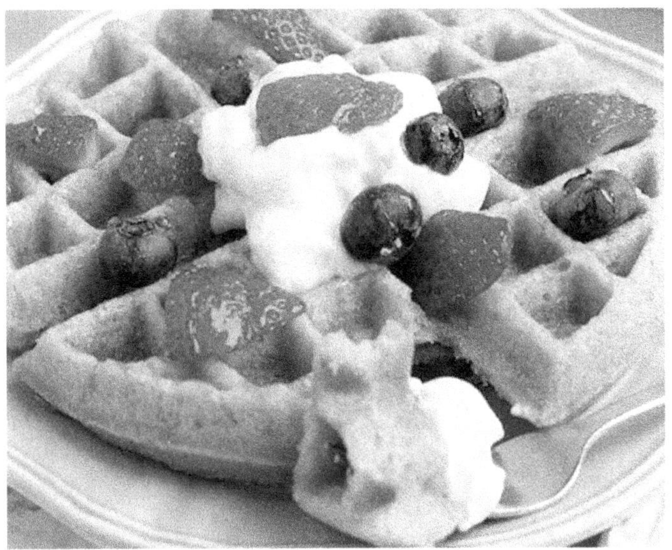

Ingredients:

- 2 cups whole grain waffle mix (low-acidity, high-fiber)
- 1 cup fresh berries (low-acidity, such as blueberries, strawberries, raspberries)
- 1 cup low-fat yogurt (1% or 2% milk fat)
- 1 tablespoon honey or maple syrup (optional, low-acidity sweeteners)

Instructions:

1. Preheat waffle iron according to package instructions.
2. Mix whole grain waffle mix with water or low-fat milk to create batter.

3. Cook waffles until crispy and golden brown.
4. Top with fresh berries and low-fat yogurt.
5. If desired, drizzle with honey or maple syrup.

8. Veggie Omelette With Whole Grain Toast

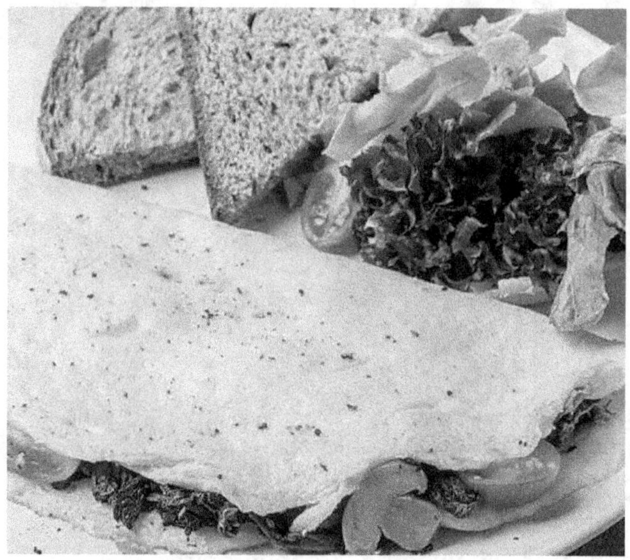

Ingredients:
- 2 eggs
- 1/2 cup mixed vegetables (low-acidity, such as bell peppers, onions, mushrooms)
- 1 tablespoon butter or non-stick cooking spray
- 2 slices whole grain bread (low-acidity, high-fiber)
- Salt and pepper to taste

Instructions:

1. In a bowl, whisk eggs and season with salt and pepper.
2. Add mixed vegetables and stir to combine.
3. Heat butter or non-stick cooking spray in a non-stick pan over medium heat.
4. Pour in egg mixture and cook until eggs are set.
5. Fold omelet in half and serve with whole grain toast.

Tips:
- Choose low-acidity vegetables like bell peppers, onions, and mushrooms.
- Use whole grain bread that is low in acidity and high in fiber.
- Cook eggs until they're fully set to avoid any acidity triggers..

9. Chia Seed Pudding With Almond Milk And Sliced Mango

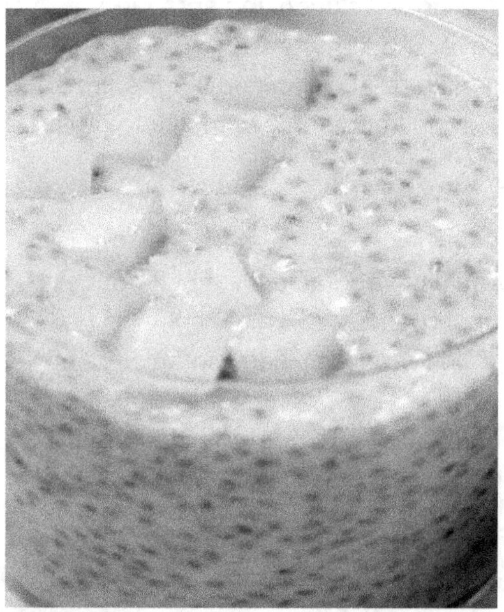

Ingredients:
- 1/2 cup chia seeds (low-acidity, high-fiber)
- 1 cup almond milk (low-acidity, low-fat)
- 1 ripe mango, sliced (low-acidity, easy to digest)
- 1 tablespoon honey or maple syrup (optional, low-acidity sweeteners)

Instructions:
1. Mix chia seeds and almond milk in a bowl.
2. Refrigerate for 2-3 hours or overnight until chia seeds absorb and form a pudding.
3. Top with sliced mango.
4. If desired, add a drizzle of honey or maple syrup.

Tips:
- Choose chia seeds as a low-acidity and high-fiber base.
- Select almond milk as a low-acidity and low-fat milk alternative.
- Opt for ripe mango for easy digestion.
- Use honey or maple syrup as low-acidity sweeteners, if desired.
- Eat slowly and mindfully to help alleviate GERD symptoms.

10. Whole Grain English Muffin With Scrambled Eggs And Spinach

Ingredients:
- 1 whole grain English muffin (low-acidity, high-fiber)
- 2 eggs
- 1/2 cup fresh spinach leaves (low-acidity, easy to digest)
- 1 tablespoon butter or non-stick cooking spray
- Salt and pepper to taste

Instructions:
1. Toast the English muffin until lightly browned.
2. In a bowl, whisk eggs and season with salt and pepper.
3. Add fresh spinach leaves and stir to combine.

4. Heat butter or non-stick cooking spray in a
non-stick pan over medium heat.
5. Pour in egg mixture and cook until eggs are set.
6. Place scrambled eggs on top of toasted English
muffin.

Tips:

- Choose a whole grain English muffin that is low in
acidity and high in fiber.
- Use fresh spinach leaves for easy digestion.
- Cook eggs until they're fully set to avoid any
acidity triggers

This recipe is a great breakfast option for a GERD
diet. The whole grain English muffin provides a
soothing and filling base, while the scrambled eggs
and spinach offer a protein-packed and
easy-to-digest complement.

11. Cottage Cheese With Sliced Cucumber And Whole Grain Crackers

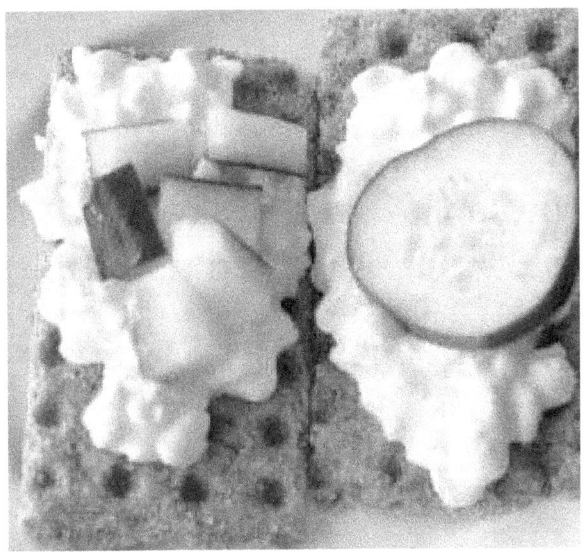

Ingredients:
- 1 cup cottage cheese (low-acidity, high-protein)
- 1/2 cup sliced cucumber (low-acidity, easy to digest)
- 5-6 whole grain crackers (low-acidity, high-fiber)
- Salt and pepper to taste

Instructions:
1. In a bowl, mix together cottage cheese and sliced cucumber.
2. Arrange whole grain crackers on a plate.
3. Top crackers with the cottage cheese and cucumber mixture.

4. Season with salt and pepper to taste.

Tips:
- Choose a low-acidity cottage cheese that is high in protein.
- Select sliced cucumber for easy digestion.
- Opt for whole grain crackers that are low in acidity and high in fiber.

12. Whole Grain Pancakes With Fresh Berries And Maple Syrup

Ingredients:
- 1 cup whole grain pancake mix (low-acidity, high-fiber)
- 1 cup fresh berries (low-acidity, such as blueberries, strawberries, raspberries)
- 2 tablespoons maple syrup (low-acidity sweetener)
- 1 cup low-fat milk (1% or 2% milk fat)
- 1 large egg
- Butter or non-stick cooking spray for greasing the pan

Instructions:
1. In a bowl, whisk together pancake mix, low-fat milk, and egg.
2. Heat a non-stick pan or griddle over medium heat.
3. Grease the pan with butter or non-stick cooking spray.

4. Pour 1/4 cup of batter onto the pan and cook until bubbles appear.
5. Flip and cook until golden brown.
6. Serve with fresh berries and maple syrup.

Tips:
- Choose a whole grain pancake mix that is low in acidity and high in fiber.
- Select fresh berries that are low in acidity and easy to digest.
- Use maple syrup as a low-acidity sweetener.
- Opt for low-fat milk and egg to avoid triggering GERD symptoms.

This recipe is a delicious and comforting breakfast option for a GERD diet. The whole grain pancakes provide a soothing and filling base, while the fresh berries offer natural sweetness and antioxidants. The maple syrup adds a touch of sweetness without triggering acidity.

13. Breakfast Burrito With Scrambled Eggs, Black Beans, And Avocado

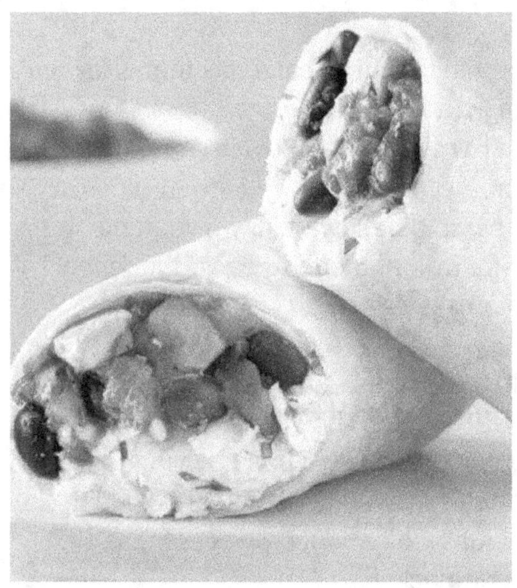

Ingredients:

- 2 scrambled eggs
- 1/2 cup cooked black beans (low-acidity, easy to digest)
- 1/2 avocado, sliced (low-acidity, soothing)
- 1 whole grain tortilla (low-acidity, high-fiber)
- Salt and pepper to taste
- Optional: salsa, sour cream, or shredded cheese (low-acidity, mild)

Instructions:

1. In a bowl, scramble eggs and season with salt
and pepper.
2. Add cooked black beans and stir to combine.
3. Add sliced avocado and stir gently.
4. Wrap mixture in a whole grain tortilla.
5. Add optional toppings, if desired.

Tips:
- Choose cooked black beans for easy digestion.
- Select ripe avocado for a soothing effect.
- Opt for a whole grain tortilla that is low in acidity
and high in fiber.
- Avoid adding high-acidity toppings like hot sauce
or citrus salsa.

This recipe is a delicious and filling breakfast option
for a GERD diet. The scrambled eggs provide a
protein-packed base, while the black beans and
avocado offer a soothing and easy-to-digest
complement. The whole grain tortilla adds fiber and
a gentle wrapping.

14. Whole Grain Bagel With Cream Cheese And Smoked Salmon

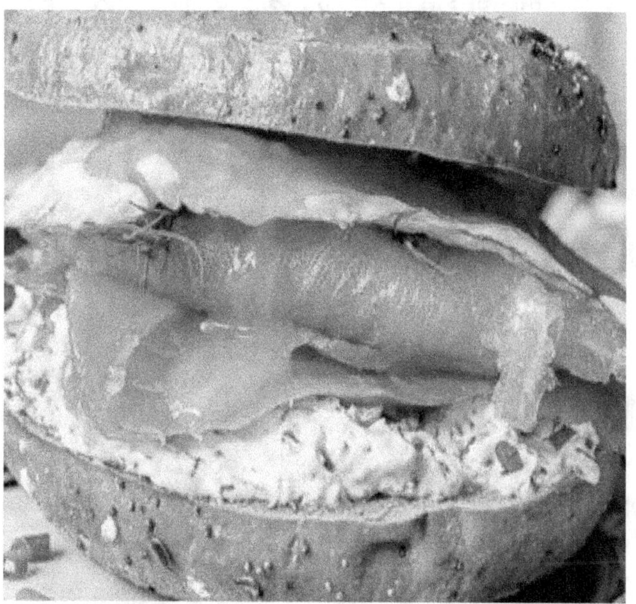

Ingredients:
- 1 whole grain bagel (low-acidity, high-fiber)
- 2 tablespoons cream cheese (low-acidity, mild)
- 2 slices smoked salmon (low-acidity, easy to digest)
- 1/4 cup sliced red onion (low-acidity, mild)
- 1/4 cup capers (low-acidity, mild)
- Salt and pepper to taste

Instructions:
1. Toast the whole grain bagel until lightly browned.

2. Spread cream cheese on the bagel.
3. Top with smoked salmon, sliced red onion, and capers.
4. Season with salt and pepper to taste.

Tips:
- Choose a whole grain bagel that is low in acidity and high in fiber.
- Select cream cheese that is low in acidity and mild.
- Opt for smoked salmon that is low in acidity and easy to digest.
- Use sliced red onion and capers in moderation, as they can trigger acidity in some individuals.
- Eat slowly and mindfully to help alleviate GERD symptoms.

This recipe is a delicious and protein-packed breakfast option for a GERD diet. The whole grain bagel provides a soothing and filling base, while the cream cheese and smoked salmon offer a creamy and easy-to-digest complement. The sliced red onion and capers add a mild and flavorful touch.

15. Whole Grain Cereal With Almond Milk And Sliced Almonds

Ingredients:
- 1 cup whole grain cereal (low-acidity, high-fiber)
- 1 cup almond milk (low-acidity, low-fat)

- 1 ounce sliced almonds (low-acidity, mild)
- Optional: 1 tablespoon honey or maple syrup
(low-acidity sweeteners)

Instructions:
1. Pour almond milk into a bowl.
2. Add whole grain cereal and stir to combine.
3. Top with sliced almonds.
4. If desired, add a drizzle of honey or maple syrup.

Tips:
- Choose a whole grain cereal that is low in acidity
and high in fiber.
- Select almond milk as a low-acidity and low-fat
milk alternative.
- Opt for sliced almonds as a low-acidity and mild
topping.
- Use honey or maple syrup as low-acidity
sweeteners, if desired.
- Eat slowly and mindfully to help alleviate GERD
symptoms.

This recipe is a quick and easy breakfast or snack
option for a GERD diet. The whole grain cereal
provides a soothing and filling base, while the
almond milk and sliced almonds offer a creamy and
mild complement. The optional honey or maple
syrup add a touch of sweetness without triggering
acidity.

16. Scrambled Eggs With Roasted Vegetables And Whole Grain Toast

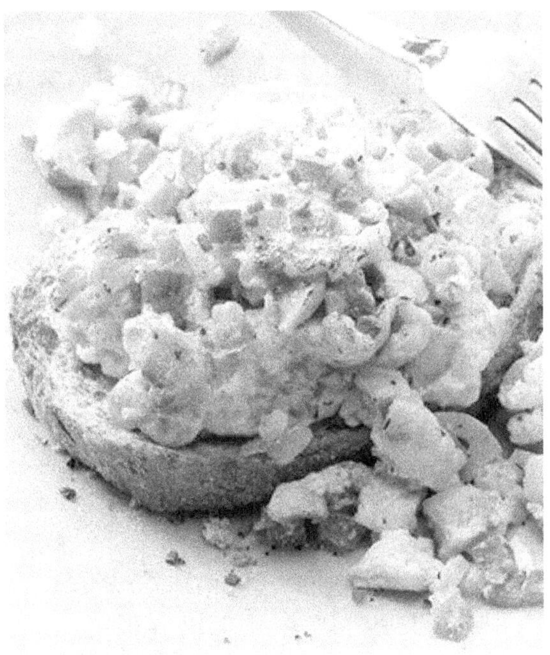

Ingredients:

- 2 eggs
- 1 cup mixed roasted vegetables (low-acidity, easy to digest)
    - Such as bell peppers, zucchini, carrots, and green beans
- 2 slices whole grain toast (low-acidity, high-fiber)
- 1 tablespoon butter or non-stick cooking spray
- Salt and pepper to taste

Instructions:
1. Preheat the oven to 400°F (200°C).
2. Toss vegetables in butter or non-stick cooking spray and roast for 20-25 minutes.
3. In a bowl, whisk eggs and season with salt and pepper.
4. Heat a non-stick pan over medium heat and add eggs.
5. Cook until eggs are set, then serve with roasted vegetables and whole grain toast.

Tips:
- Choose low-acidity vegetables that are easy to digest.
- Select whole grain toast that is low in acidity and high in fiber.
- Cook eggs until they're fully set to avoid any acidity triggers.

This recipe is a delicious and balanced breakfast option for a GERD diet. The scrambled eggs provide a protein-packed base, while the roasted vegetables offer a flavorful and easy-to-digest complement. The whole grain toast adds fiber and a soothing element.

17. Whole Grain Muffin With Fresh Berries And Yogurt

Ingredients:
- 1 whole grain muffin (low-acidity, high-fiber)

- 1/2 cup fresh berries (low-acidity, easy to digest)
    - Such as blueberries, strawberries, or raspberries
- 1/2 cup low-fat yogurt (low-acidity, soothing)
- 1 tablespoon honey or maple syrup (optional, low-acidity sweeteners)

Instructions:
1. Toast the whole grain muffin until lightly browned.
2. Top with fresh berries and low-fat yogurt.
3. If desired, drizzle with honey or maple syrup.

Tips:
- Choose a whole grain muffin that is low in acidity and high in fiber.
- Select fresh berries that are low in acidity and easy to digest.
- Opt for low-fat yogurt that is low in acidity and soothing.
- Use honey or maple syrup as low-acidity sweeteners, if desired.

This recipe is a delicious and soothing breakfast option for a GERD diet. The whole grain muffin provides a filling base, while the fresh berries offer natural sweetness and antioxidants. The low-fat yogurt adds a creamy and calming element.

18. Breakfast Quesadillas With Scrambled Eggs,Black Beans And Avocado

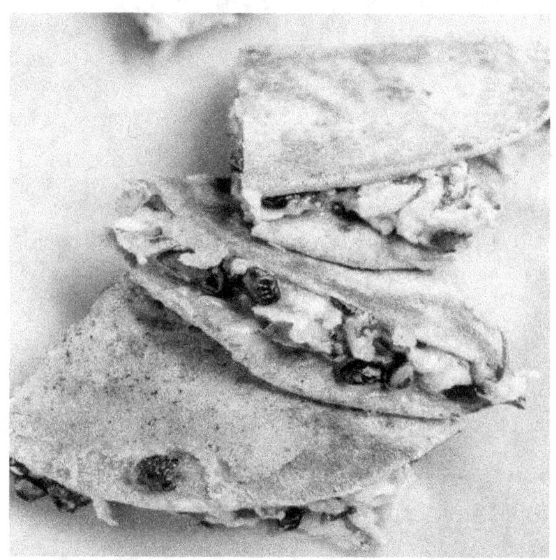

Ingredients:
- 2 whole grain tortillas (low-acidity, high-fiber)
- 2 scrambled eggs
- 1/2 cup cooked black beans (low-acidity, easy to digest)
- 1/2 avocado, sliced (low-acidity, soothing)
- 1 tablespoon olive oil
- Salt and pepper to taste
- Optional: salsa, sour cream, or shredded cheese (low-acidity, mild)

Instructions:

1. In a bowl, scramble eggs and season with salt
and pepper.
2. Add cooked black beans and stir to combine.
3. Heat olive oil in a non-stick pan over medium
heat.
4. Place a tortilla in the pan and add egg mixture
and avocado slices.
5. Fold tortilla in half and cook until crispy and
melted.
6. Repeat with a second tortilla and fill.
7. Cut into wedges and serve with optional
toppings.

Tips:
- Choose whole grain tortillas that are low in acidity
and high in fiber.
- Select cooked black beans that are easy to digest.
- Opt for ripe avocado for a soothing effect.
- Use mild toppings like salsa, sour cream, or
shredded cheese, if desired.

This recipe is a delicious and filling breakfast option
for a GERD diet. The scrambled eggs provide a
protein-packed base, while the black beans and
avocado offer a soothing and easy-to-digest
complement. The whole grain tortillas add fiber and
a gentle wrapping.

19. Whole Grain Toast With Almond Butter And Sliced Banana

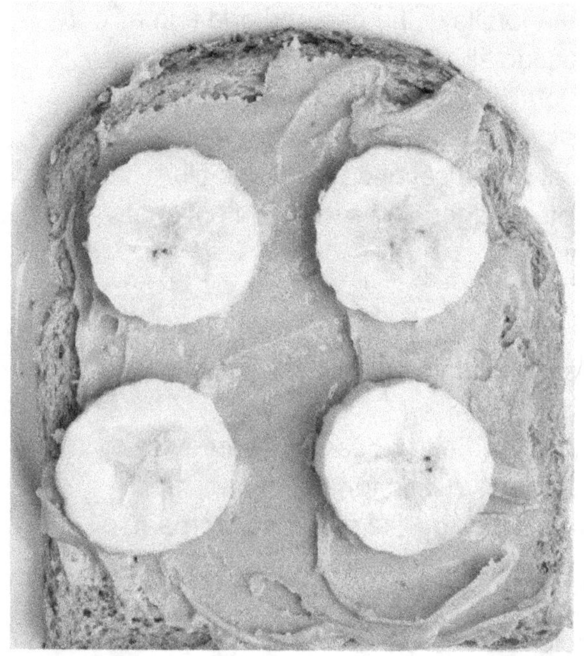

Ingredients:
- 2 slices whole grain bread (low-acidity, high-fiber)
- 2 tablespoons almond butter (low-acidity, soothing)
- 1 ripe banana, sliced (low-acidity, easy to digest)
- Pinch of salt

Instructions:
1. Toast whole grain bread until lightly browned.
2. Spread almond butter on each slice.

3. Top with sliced banana.

4. Sprinkle with a pinch of salt.

Tips:

- Choose whole grain bread that is low in acidity and high in fiber.

- Select almond butter that is low in acidity and soothing.

- Opt for a ripe banana that is easy to digest.

This recipe is a delicious and soothing breakfast or snack option for a GERD diet. The whole grain toast provides a filling base, while the almond butter offers a creamy and calming element. The sliced banana adds natural sweetness and easy digestion.

20. Green Smoothie With Spinach,Almond Milk,And Chia Seeds

Ingredients:

- 2 cups fresh spinach leaves (low-acidity, easy to digest)

- 1 cup almond milk (low-acidity, low-fat)

- 1 tablespoon chia seeds (low-acidity, soothing)

- 1/2 banana, sliced (low-acidity, easy to digest)

- 1/2 cup frozen pineapple (low-acidity, sweet)

- 1 tablespoon honey or maple syrup (optional, low-acidity sweeteners)

Instructions:
1. Add all ingredients to a blender and blend until smooth.
2. Taste and adjust sweetness with honey or maple syrup, if desired.
3. Pour into a glass and serve immediately.

Tips:
- Choose fresh spinach leaves that are low in acidity and easy to digest.
- Select almond milk that is low in acidity and low-fat.
- Opt for chia seeds that are low in acidity and soothing.
- Use a ripe banana and frozen pineapple for natural sweetness and easy digestion.
- Eat slowly and mindfully to help alleviate GERD symptoms.

This recipe is a nutritious and filling breakfast or snack option for a GERD diet. The spinach provides a boost of antioxidants, while the almond milk and chia seeds offer a creamy and soothing element. The banana and pineapple add natural sweetness and easy digestion.

Tasty Lunch Recipes

1. Grilled Chicken Breast With Roasted Vegetables

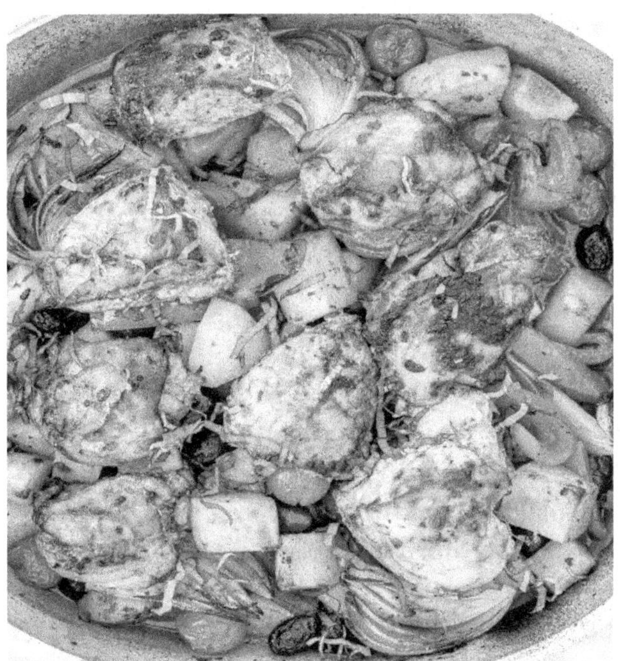

Ingredients:
- 4 boneless, skinless chicken breasts (low-acidity, lean protein)
- 2 tablespoons olive oil (low-acidity, healthy fat)
- 1 teaspoon dried thyme (low-acidity, soothing herb)
- 1 teaspoon garlic powder (low-acidity, mild flavor)
- Salt and pepper to taste

- 4 cups mixed roasted vegetables (low-acidity, easy to digest)
    - Such as zucchini, bell peppers, carrots, and green beans

Instructions:
1. Preheat the grill to medium-high heat.
2. In a small bowl, whisk together olive oil, thyme, garlic powder, salt, and pepper.
3. Brush mixture on both sides of chicken breasts.
4. Grill chicken for 5-6 minutes per side or until cooked through.
5. Toss vegetables in olive oil, salt, and pepper.
6. Spread on a baking sheet and roast in the oven at 400°F (200°C) for 20-25 minutes or until tender.
7. Serve chicken with roasted vegetables.

Tips:
- Choose lean protein like chicken breast to reduce fat and acidity.
- Select low-acidity vegetables that are easy to digest.
- Use herbs like thyme and garlic powder for flavor instead of acidic spices.

This recipe is a delicious and balanced lunch option for a GERD diet. The grilled chicken provides a lean protein source, while the roasted vegetables offer a flavorful and easy-to-digest complement.

2. Whole Grain Pita With Hummus,Cucumber And Bell Peppers

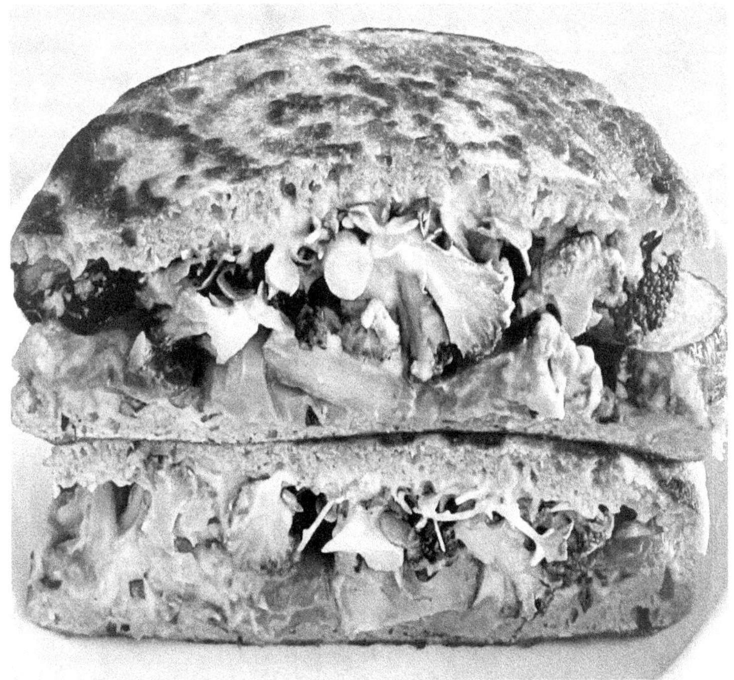

Ingredients:
- 1 whole grain pita bread (low-acidity, high-fiber)
- 1/2 cup hummus (low-acidity, soothing)
- 1/2 cucumber, sliced (low-acidity, easy to digest)
- 1/2 bell pepper, sliced (low-acidity, sweet)
- Salt and pepper to taste
- Optional: 1/4 cup sliced cherry tomatoes
(low-acidity, sweet)

Instructions:
1. Spread hummus on the whole grain pita bread.
2. Top with sliced cucumber and bell pepper.
3. Add cherry tomatoes, if desired.
4. Season with salt and pepper to taste.
5. Serve and enjoy!

Tips:
- Choose whole grain pita bread for a low-acidity and high-fiber base.
- Select hummus that is low in acidity and soothing.
- Opt for cucumber and bell pepper slices that are easy to digest.
- Add cherry tomatoes for a burst of sweetness and flavor.

This recipe is a tasty and refreshing lunch option for a GERD diet. The whole grain pita provides a filling base, while the hummus offers a creamy and soothing element. The cucumber and bell pepper add crunch and flavor, and the cherry tomatoes provide a sweet and tangy touch.

3. Lentil Soup with Whole Grain Bread

Ingredients:
- 1 cup dried green or brown lentils (low-acidity, easy to digest)
- 4 cups vegetable broth (low-acidity, soothing)
- 1 onion, chopped (low-acidity, mild flavor)

- 2 cloves garlic, minced (low-acidity, mild flavor)
- 1 carrot, chopped (low-acidity, sweet)
- 1 celery stalk, chopped (low-acidity, mild flavor)
- 1 can diced tomatoes (low-acidity, sweet)
- 1 teaspoon dried thyme (low-acidity, soothing herb)
- Salt and pepper to taste
- 2 slices whole grain bread (low-acidity, high-fiber)

Instructions:
1. In a pot, sauté onion, garlic, carrot, and celery in olive oil until tender.
2. Add lentils, vegetable broth, diced tomatoes, and thyme.
3. Bring to a boil, then simmer for 30-40 minutes or until lentils are tender.
4. Season with salt and pepper to taste.
5. Serve with whole grain bread.

Tips:
- Choose low-acidity lentils that are easy to digest.
- Select vegetable broth that is low in acidity and soothing.
- Opt for mild flavors like onion, garlic, carrot, and celery.
- Add diced tomatoes for a sweet and tangy flavor.
- Use thyme for a soothing and calming effect.

This recipe is a comforting and nutritious lunch option for a GERD diet. The lentil soup provides a filling and easy-to-digest base, while the whole grain bread offers a soothing and fiber-rich complement.

4. Quinoa Salad With Grilled Turkey,Avocado And Cherry Tomatoes

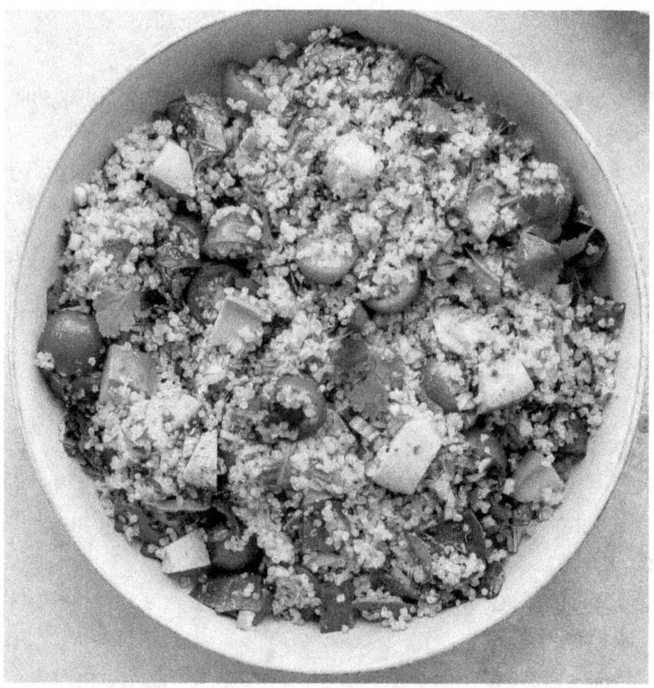

Ingredients:
- 1 cup cooked quinoa (low-acidity, easy to digest)
- 4 oz grilled turkey breast (low-acidity, lean protein)
- 1 ripe avocado, diced (low-acidity, soothing)
- 1 cup cherry tomatoes, halved (low-acidity, sweet)

- 1/4 cup chopped fresh parsley (low-acidity, mild flavor)
- 2 tablespoons olive oil (low-acidity, healthy fat)
- 1 tablespoon lemon juice (low-acidity, mild flavor)
- Salt and pepper to taste

Instructions:
1. In a bowl, combine cooked quinoa, grilled turkey, avocado, cherry tomatoes, and parsley.
2. In a small bowl, whisk together olive oil and lemon juice.
3. Pour dressing over quinoa mixture and toss to combine.
4. Season with salt and pepper to taste.
5. Serve and enjoy!

Tips:
- Choose cooked quinoa for a low-acidity and easy-to-digest base.
- Select grilled turkey breast for a lean protein source.
- Opt for ripe avocado for a soothing and creamy element.
- Add cherry tomatoes for a sweet and tangy flavor.
- Use fresh parsley for a mild and fresh flavor.

This recipe is a delicious and nutritious lunch option for a GERD diet. The quinoa salad provides a filling and easy-to-digest base, while the grilled turkey offers a lean protein source. The avocado adds a soothing and creamy element, and the cherry tomatoes provide a sweet and tangy flavor.

5. Baked Cod With Sweet Potato And Green Beans

Ingredients:
- 4 cod filets (low-acidity, lean protein)
- 2 large sweet potatoes, peeled and cubed (low-acidity, easy to digest)
- 1 pound fresh green beans, trimmed (low-acidity, easy to digest)
- 2 tablespoons olive oil (low-acidity, healthy fat)
- 1 teaspoon dried thyme (low-acidity, soothing herb)
- Salt and pepper to taste

Instructions:
1. Preheat the oven to 400°F (200°C).
2. Line a baking sheet with parchment paper.
3. Place cod filets on the baking sheet.
4. Drizzle with olive oil and sprinkle with thyme.
5. Bake for 12-15 minutes or until cod is cooked through.
6. Toss sweet potatoes and green beans in olive oil, salt, and pepper.
7. Spread on a separate baking sheet and roast for 20-25 minutes or until tender.
8. Serve cod with roasted sweet potatoes and green beans.

Tips:
- Choose cod filets for a low-acidity and lean protein source.

- Select sweet potatoes and green beans for easy-to-digest and low-acidity vegetables.
- Use olive oil for a healthy fat and thyme for a soothing herb.

This recipe is a delicious and balanced dinner option for a GERD diet. The baked cod provides a lean protein source, while the sweet potatoes and green beans offer easy-to-digest and low-acidity vegetables.

6. Veggie Wrap With Whole Grain Wrap,Eggplant,And Red Pepper

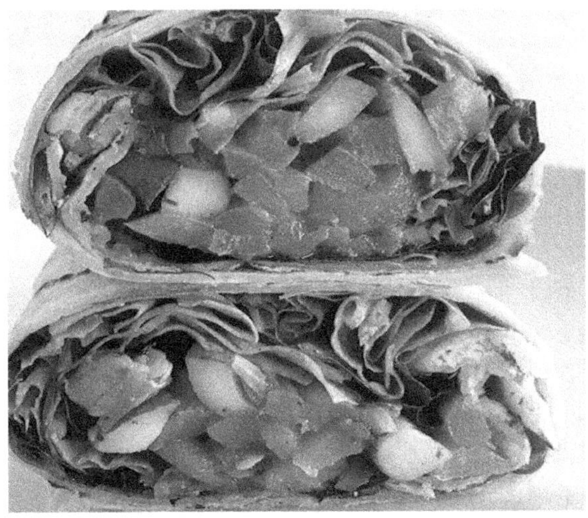

Ingredients:
- 1 whole grain wrap (low-acidity, high-fiber)
- 1 medium eggplant, sliced (low-acidity, easy to digest)

- 1 medium red pepper, sliced (low-acidity, sweet)
- 1/4 cup hummus (low-acidity, soothing)
- 1/4 cup mixed greens (low-acidity, mild flavor)
- Salt and pepper to taste

Instructions:
1. Preheat a grill or grill pan to medium heat.
2. Brush eggplant and red pepper slices with olive oil and season with salt and pepper.
3. Grill for 3-4 minutes per side or until tender.
4. Spread hummus on the whole grain wrap.
5. Add grilled eggplant and red pepper slices.
6. Top with mixed greens.
7. Roll up and slice in half.

Tips:
- Choose a whole grain wrap for a low-acidity and high-fiber base.
- Select eggplant and red pepper for low-acidity and easy-to-digest vegetables.
- Use hummus for a soothing and creamy element.
- Add mixed greens for a mild and fresh flavor.

This recipe is a tasty and healthy lunch option for a GERD diet. The whole grain wrap provides a filling base, while the grilled eggplant and red pepper offer a flavorful and easy-to-digest complement. The hummus adds a soothing and creamy element, and the mixed greens provide a fresh and mild flavor.

7. Chicken And Vegetable Stir-Fry With Brown Rice

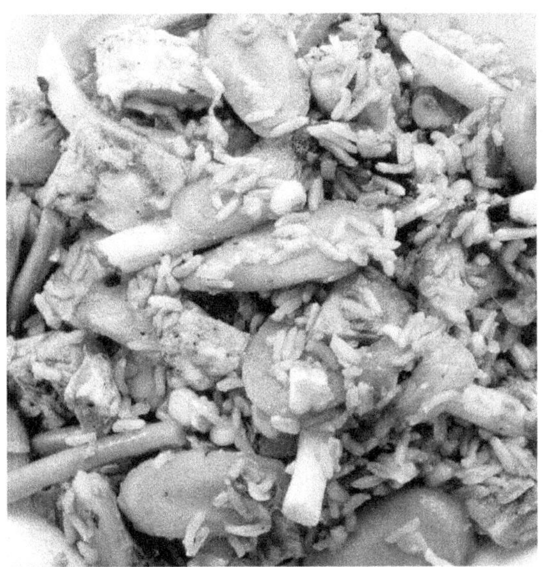

Ingredients:
- 1 pound boneless, skinless chicken breast (low-acidity, lean protein)
- 2 cups mixed vegetables (low-acidity, easy to digest)
    - Such as bell peppers, carrots, broccoli, and snap peas
- 2 tablespoons olive oil (low-acidity, healthy fat)
- 2 cloves garlic, minced (low-acidity, mild flavor)
- 1 cup cooked brown rice (low-acidity, easy to digest)
- Salt and pepper to taste

Instructions:

1. Cook brown rice according to package
instructions.
2. In a large skillet or wok, heat olive oil over
medium-high heat.
3. Add chicken and cook until browned and cooked
through.
4. Add mixed vegetables and garlic and stir-fry until
tender.
5. Serve chicken and vegetable mixture over brown
rice.

Tips:
- Choose lean protein like chicken breast to reduce
fat and acidity.
- Select low-acidity vegetables that are easy to
digest.
- Use olive oil for a healthy fat and garlic for a mild
flavor.

This recipe is a flavorful and balanced dinner option
for a GERD diet. The chicken and vegetable stir-fry
provides a lean protein source and easy-to-digest
vegetables, while the brown rice offers a soothing
and fiber-rich complement.

8. Whole Grain Crackers With Marinara Sauce And Sauteed Spinach

Ingredients:
- 1 box whole grain crackers (low-acidity, high-fiber)

- 1 cup Marinara sauce (low-acidity, mild flavor)
- 1 cup fresh spinach leaves (low-acidity, easy to digest)
- 1 tablespoon olive oil (low-acidity, healthy fat)
- Salt and pepper to taste

Instructions:
1. Preheat a skillet over medium heat.
2. Add olive oil and sauté spinach until wilted.
3. Spread Marinara sauce on whole grain crackers.
4. Top with sautéed spinach.
5. Season with salt and pepper to taste.

Tips:
- Choose whole grain crackers for a low-acidity and high-fiber base.
- Select Marinara sauce with low-acidity and mild flavor.
- Use fresh spinach for a low-acidity and easy-to-digest vegetable.

This recipe is a tasty and healthy snack option for a GERD diet. The whole grain crackers provide a filling base, while the Marinara sauce offers a mild and slightly sweet flavor. The sautéed spinach adds a nutritious and easy-to-digest element.

9. Grilled Chicken And Quinoa Bowl With Roasted Vegetables

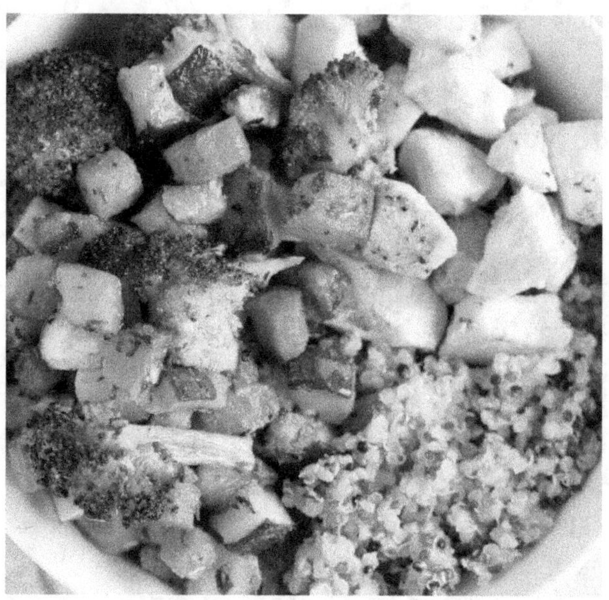

Ingredients:
- 1 pound boneless, skinless chicken breast (low-acidity, lean protein)
- 1 cup cooked quinoa (low-acidity, easy to digest)
- 2 cups mixed roasted vegetables (low-acidity, easy to digest)
    - Such as zucchini, bell peppers, carrots, and green beans
- 2 tablespoons olive oil (low-acidity, healthy fat)
- Salt and pepper to taste

Instructions:
1. Grill chicken breast until cooked through.

2. Cook quinoa according to package instructions.
3. Toss vegetables in olive oil and roast in the oven until tender.
4. Assemble bowl with grilled chicken, quinoa, and roasted vegetables.
5. Season with salt and pepper to taste.

Tips:
- Choose lean protein like chicken breast to reduce fat and acidity.
- Select quinoa for a low-acidity and easy-to-digest grain.
- Opt for low-acidity vegetables that are easy to digest.
- Use olive oil for a healthy fat.

This recipe is a nutritious and balanced meal option for a GERD diet. The grilled chicken provides a lean protein source, while the quinoa offers a soothing and fiber-rich complement. The roasted vegetables add a flavorful and easy-to-digest element.

10. Turkey And Avocado Wrap With Mixed Greens

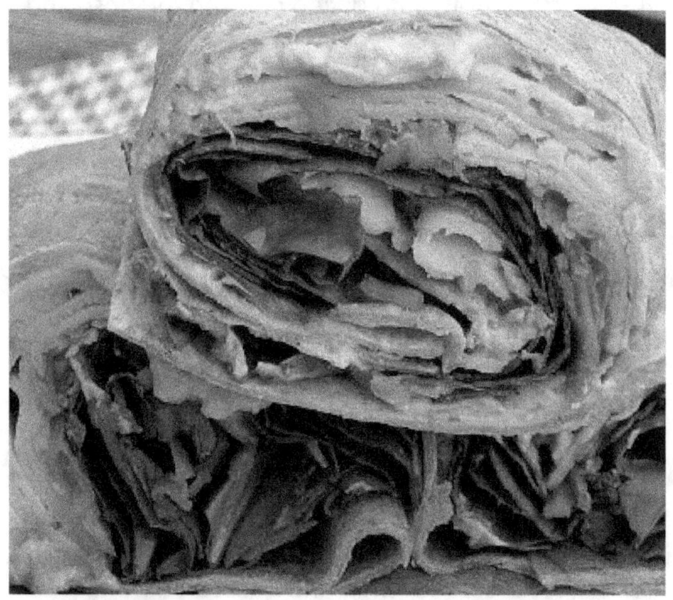

Ingredients:
- 1 slice whole grain wrap (low-acidity, high-fiber)
- 2 oz sliced turkey breast (low-acidity, lean protein)
- 1/2 avocado, sliced (low-acidity, soothing)
- 1 cup mixed greens (low-acidity, mild flavor)
- 1/4 cup sliced cucumber (low-acidity, easy to digest)
- 1/4 cup sliced bell peppers (low-acidity, sweet)

Instructions:
1. Lay wrap flat and arrange ingredients in the center.

2. Add sliced turkey, avocado, mixed greens, cucumber, and bell peppers.
3. Fold bottom half up and fold in sides.
4. Roll up wrap tightly.
5. Slice in half and serve.

Tips:
- Choose whole grain wrap for a low-acidity and high-fiber base.
- Select sliced turkey breast for a lean protein source.
- Use avocado for a soothing and creamy element.
- Add mixed greens for a mild and fresh flavor.
- Include cucumber and bell peppers for easy-to-digest vegetables.

This recipe is a tasty and healthy lunch option for a GERD diet. The whole grain wrap provides a filling base, while the turkey and avocado offer a lean protein source and soothing element. The mixed greens, cucumber, and bell peppers add a fresh and easy-to-digest complement.

11. Lentil And Vegetable Curry With Brown Rice

Ingredients:
- 1 cup red or green lentils (low-acidity, easy to digest)
- 2 cups water (low-acidity, hydrating)
- 1 tablespoon olive oil (low-acidity, healthy fat)

- 1 onion, chopped (low-acidity, mild flavor)
- 2 cloves garlic, minced (low-acidity, mild flavor)
- 1 carrot, chopped (low-acidity, easy to digest)
- 1 zucchini, chopped (low-acidity, easy to digest)
- 1 cup mixed vegetables (low-acidity, easy to digest)
- 1 teaspoon curry powder (low-acidity, mild flavor)
- Salt and pepper to taste
- 1 cup cooked brown rice (low-acidity, easy to digest)

Instructions:
1. Cook lentils in water until tender.
2. In a large skillet, heat olive oil over medium heat.
3. Add onion, garlic, carrot, zucchini, and mixed vegetables.
4. Cook until vegetables are tender.
5. Stir in curry powder and cooked lentils.
6. Season with salt and pepper to taste.
7. Serve over brown rice.

Tips:
- Choose low-acidity lentils and vegetables to reduce acidity.
- Use olive oil for a healthy fat and curry powder for a mild flavor.

This recipe is a flavorful and nutritious meal option for a GERD diet. The lentil and vegetable curry provides a low-acidity and easy-to-digest protein source, while the brown rice offers a soothing and fiber-rich complement.

12. Grilled Salmon With Roasted Asparagus And Quinoa

Ingredients:
- 6 oz salmon filet (low-acidity, lean protein)
- 1 pound fresh asparagus (low-acidity, easy to digest)

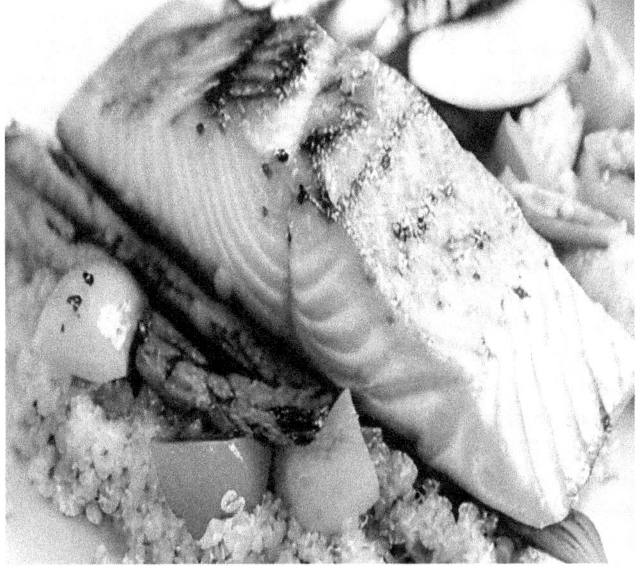

- 1 cup cooked quinoa (low-acidity, easy to digest)
- 2 tablespoons olive oil (low-acidity, healthy fat)
- Salt and pepper to taste

Instructions:
1. Preheat the grill to medium-high heat.
2. Season salmon with salt and pepper.

3. Grill for 4-6 minutes per side or until cooked through.
4. Toss asparagus in olive oil and roast in the oven until tender.
5. Cook quinoa according to package instructions.
6. Serve salmon with roasted asparagus and quinoa.

Tips:
- Choose lean protein like salmon to reduce fat and acidity.
- Select low-acidity asparagus and quinoa for easy digestion.
- Use olive oil for a healthy fat.

This recipe is a delicious and balanced meal option for a GERD diet. The grilled salmon provides a lean protein source, while the roasted asparagus and quinoa offer easy-to-digest vegetables and a soothing grain.

13. Veggies And Hummus Sandwich On Whole Grain Bread

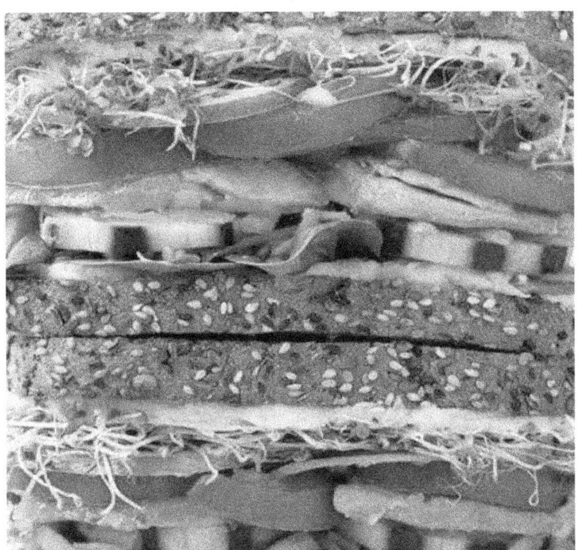

Ingredients:
- 2 slices whole grain bread (low-acidity, high-fiber)
- 1/4 cup hummus (low-acidity, soothing)
- 1 cup mixed vegetables (low-acidity, easy to digest)
    - Such as cucumber, bell peppers, carrots, and spinach
- 1 tablespoon olive oil (low-acidity, healthy fat)
- Salt and pepper to taste

Instructions:
1. Spread hummus on one slice of bread.
2. Add mixed vegetables.
3. Drizzle with olive oil.

4. Top with a second slice of bread.
5. Serve and enjoy!

Tips:
- Choose whole grain bread for a low-acidity and high-fiber base.
- Select low-acidity vegetables that are easy to digest.
- Use hummus for a soothing and creamy element.

This recipe is a tasty and healthy snack option for a GERD diet. The whole grain bread provides a filling base, while the hummus and mixed vegetables offer a soothing and easy-to-digest complement.

14. Chicken And Mushroom Risotto With Whole Grain Rice

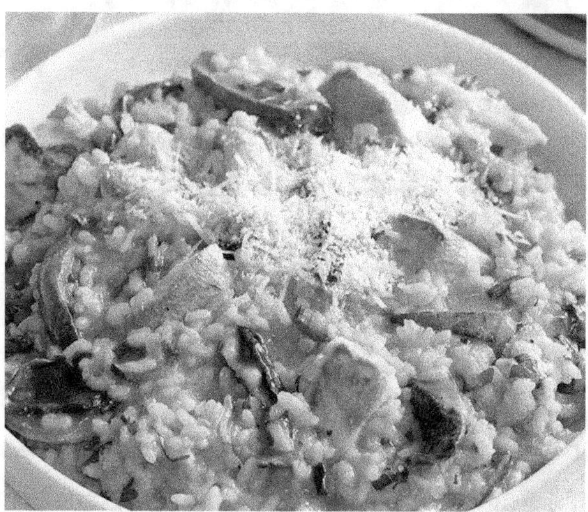

Ingredients:
- 1 pound boneless, skinless chicken breast (low-acidity, lean protein)
- 1 cup mixed mushrooms (low-acidity, easy to digest)
- 1 cup whole grain rice (low-acidity, high-fiber)
- 4 cups vegetable broth (low-acidity, hydrating)
- 1 tablespoon olive oil (low-acidity, healthy fat)
- 1 teaspoon dried thyme (low-acidity, soothing herb)
- Salt and pepper to taste

Instructions:
1. Cook whole grain rice according to package instructions.
2. In a large skillet, heat olive oil over medium heat.
3. Add chicken and cook until browned and cooked through.
4. Add mushrooms and cook until tender.
5. Add vegetable broth, one cup at a time, stirring continuously.
6. Stir in cooked rice and thyme.
7. Season with salt and pepper to taste.

Tips:
- Choose lean protein like chicken breast to reduce fat and acidity.
- Select low-acidity mushrooms and whole grain rice for easy digestion.
- Use olive oil for a healthy fat and thyme for a soothing herb.

This recipe is a creamy and comforting meal option for a GERD diet. The chicken and mushroom risotto provides a lean protein source and easy-to-digest vegetables, while the whole grain rice offers a soothing and fiber-rich complement.

15. Whole Grain Sushi Rolls With Cucumber And Avocado

Ingredients:
- 1 cup cooked whole grain rice (low-acidity, high-fiber)
- 1/2 avocado, sliced (low-acidity, soothing)
- 1/2 cucumber, sliced (low-acidity, easy to digest)
- 1 sheet whole grain nori seaweed (low-acidity, high-fiber)
- 1 tablespoon rice vinegar (low-acidity, mild flavor)

Instructions:
1. Prepare whole grain rice according to package instructions.
2. Mix rice vinegar into cooked rice.
3. Lay nori sheet flat.
4. Spread rice mixture onto nori, leaving a small border.
5. Add avocado and cucumber slices.
6. Roll up sushi and slice into pieces.

Tips:
- Choose whole grain rice and nori for a low-acidity and high-fiber base.

- Select low-acidity avocado and cucumber for easy digestion.
- Use rice vinegar for a mild flavor.

This recipe is a refreshing and healthy snack option for a GERD diet. The whole grain sushi rolls provide a soothing and fiber-rich base, while the avocado and cucumber offer a creamy and easy-to-digest complement.

16. Grilled Chicken And Vegetable Skewers With Quinoa

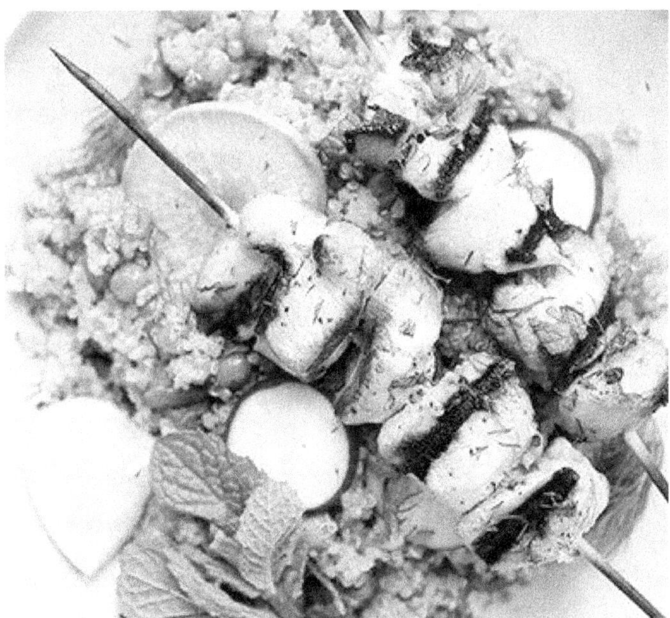

Ingredients:

- 1 pound boneless, skinless chicken breast
(low-acidity, lean protein)
- 1 cup mixed vegetables (low-acidity, easy to
digest)
    - Such as bell peppers, zucchini, cherry
tomatoes, and onions
- 1 cup cooked quinoa (low-acidity, high-fiber)
- 2 tablespoons olive oil (low-acidity, healthy fat)
- 1 tablespoon lemon juice (low-acidity, mild flavor)
- Salt and pepper to taste

Instructions:
1. Preheat the grill to medium-high heat.
2. Thread chicken and vegetables onto skewers.
3. Brush with olive oil and season with salt, pepper,
and lemon juice.
4. Grill for 10-12 minutes or until chicken is cooked
through.
5. Serve with quinoa.

Tips:
- Choose lean protein like chicken breast to reduce
fat and acidity.
- Select low-acidity vegetables that are easy to
digest.
- Use olive oil for a healthy fat and lemon juice for a
mild flavor.

This recipe is a flavorful and nutritious meal option
for a GERD diet. The grilled chicken and vegetable
skewers provide a lean protein source and

easy-to-digest vegetables, while the quinoa offers a soothing and fiber-rich complement.

17. Spinach And Feta Stuffed Chicken Breast With Roasted Vegetables

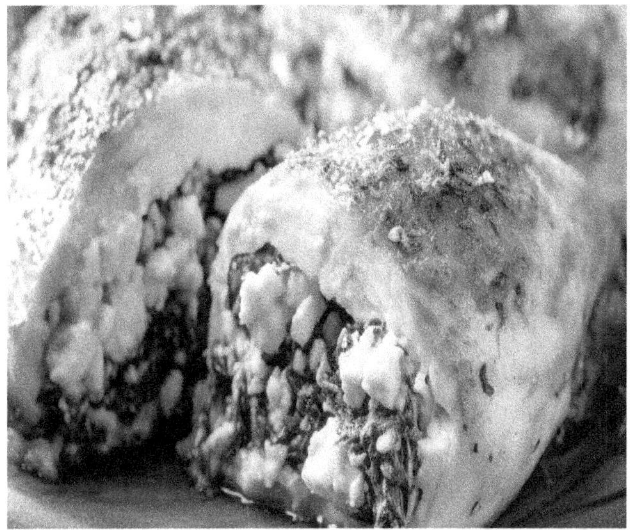

Ingredients:
- 4 boneless, skinless chicken breasts (low-acidity, lean protein)
- 1 cup fresh spinach (low-acidity, easy to digest)
- 1/2 cup crumbled feta cheese (low-acidity, mild flavor)
- 1 cup mixed roasted vegetables (low-acidity, easy to digest)
    - Such as Brussels sprouts, carrots, and sweet potatoes

- 2 tablespoons olive oil (low-acidity, healthy fat)
- Salt and pepper to taste

Instructions:
1. Preheat the oven to 375°F (190°C).
2. Stuff each chicken breast with spinach and feta cheese.
3. Place on a baking sheet with roasted vegetables.
4. Drizzle with olive oil and season with salt and pepper.
5. Bake for 30-35 minutes or until chicken is cooked through.

Tips:
- Choose lean protein like chicken breast to reduce fat and acidity.
- Select low-acidity spinach and feta cheese for easy digestion.
- Use olive oil for a healthy fat and roasted vegetables for a soothing complement.

This recipe is a flavorful and nutritious meal option for a GERD diet. The spinach and feta stuffed chicken breast provides a lean protein source and easy-to-digest ingredients, while the roasted vegetables offer a soothing and fiber-rich complement.

18. Whole Grain Pita with Falafel,Lettuce And Tomato

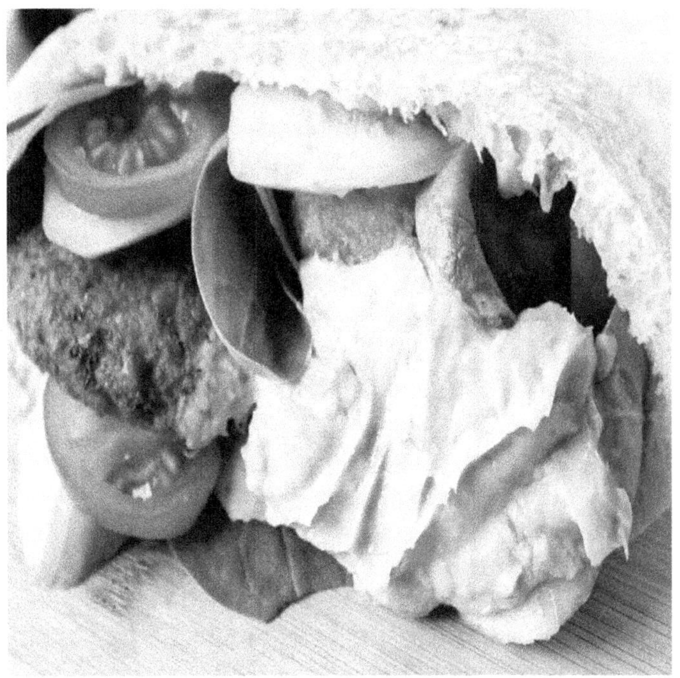

Ingredients:
- 1 whole grain pita bread (low-acidity, high-fiber)
- 4 falafel patties (low-acidity, made with chickpeas)
- 1 cup shredded lettuce (low-acidity, easy to digest)
- 1 cup sliced tomatoes (low-acidity, easy to digest)
- 1/4 cup tahini sauce (low-acidity, made with sesame seeds)
- Salt and pepper to taste

Instructions:

1. Toast pita bread.
2. Fill with falafel patties, lettuce, tomatoes, and tahini sauce.
3. Serve and enjoy.

Tips:
- Choose whole grain pita bread for a low-acidity and high-fiber base.
- Select falafel made with chickpeas for a low-acidity protein source.
- Use shredded lettuce and sliced tomatoes for easy digestion.
- Opt for tahini sauce made with sesame seeds for a low-acidity condiment.
- Eat slowly and mindfully to help alleviate GERD symptoms.

This recipe is a tasty and healthy meal option for a GERD diet. The whole grain pita provides a soothing base, while the falafel, lettuce, and tomato offer a flavorful and easy-to-digest filling.

19. Shrimp And Vegetable Stir-Fry With Brown Rice

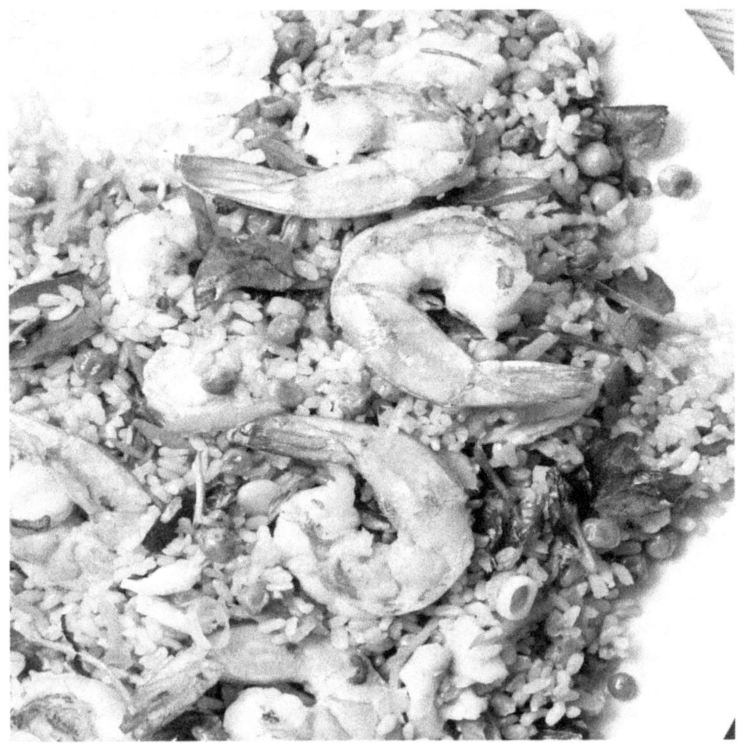

Ingredients:
- 1 pound large shrimp (low-acidity, lean protein)
- 1 cup mixed vegetables (low-acidity, easy to digest)
    - Such as bell peppers, carrots, and snow peas
- 2 tablespoons olive oil (low-acidity, healthy fat)
- 1 cup cooked brown rice (low-acidity, high-fiber)
- 2 cloves garlic, minced (low-acidity, mild flavor)
- 1 teaspoon grated ginger (low-acidity, soothing)

- Salt and pepper to taste

Instructions:
1. Cook brown rice according to package instructions.
2. In a large skillet, heat olive oil over medium-high heat.
3. Add shrimp, vegetables, garlic, and ginger.
4. Stir-fry until shrimp are pink and vegetables are tender.
5. Serve over brown rice.

Tips:
- Choose lean protein like shrimp to reduce fat and acidity.
- Select low-acidity vegetables that are easy to digest.
- Use olive oil for a healthy fat and garlic and ginger for mild flavors.

This recipe is a flavorful and nutritious meal option for a GERD diet. The shrimp and vegetable stir-fry provides a lean protein source and easy-to-digest vegetables, while the brown rice offers a soothing and fiber-rich complement.

20. Grilled Turkey And Cheese Sandwich In Whole Grain Bread With Carrot Sticks

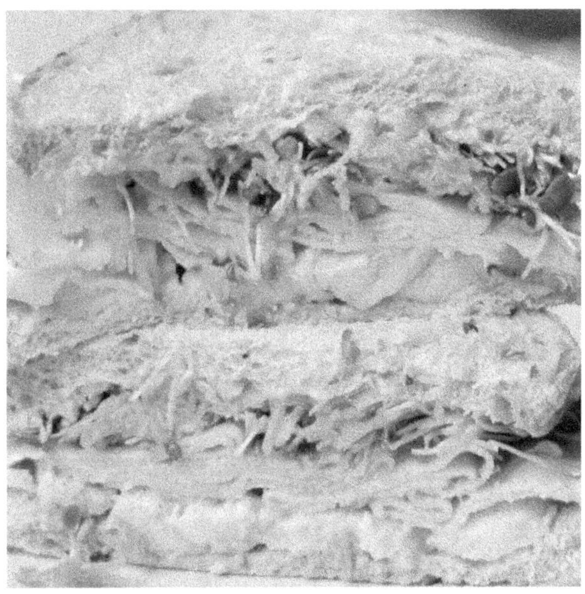

Ingredients:
- 2 slices whole grain bread (low-acidity, high-fiber)
- 2 oz sliced turkey breast (low-acidity, lean protein)
- 1 oz sliced cheese (low-acidity, mild flavor)
- 1/4 cup sliced carrot sticks (low-acidity, easy to digest)
- 1 tablespoon olive oil (low-acidity, healthy fat)
- Salt and pepper to taste

Instructions:
1. Preheat the grill or grill pan to medium heat.

2. Place turkey and cheese between whole grain
bread slices.
3. Grill until bread is toasted and cheese is melted.
4. Serve with carrot sticks and olive oil for dipping.

Tips:
- Choose whole grain bread for a low-acidity and
high-fiber base.
- Select lean protein like turkey breast to reduce fat
and acidity.
- Opt for mild cheese for a low-acidity filling.
- Include carrot sticks for a crunchy and
easy-to-digest snack.
- Use olive oil for a healthy fat and eat slowly to
alleviate GERD symptoms.

This recipe is a satisfying and healthy meal option
for a GERD diet. The grilled turkey and cheese
sandwich provides a lean protein source and
easy-to-digest filling, while the whole grain bread
and carrot sticks offer a soothing and fiber-rich
complement. Enjoy

Mouth-Watering Dinner Recipes

1. Grilled Salmon With Roasted Vegetables

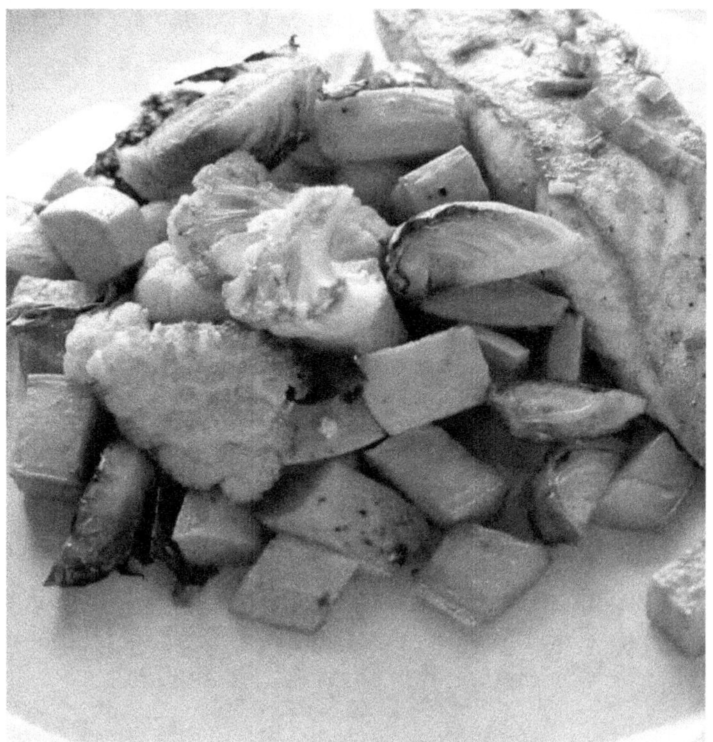

Ingredients:
- 6 oz salmon filet (wild-caught Alaskan or Atlantic)
- 2 cups mixed vegetables (such as Brussels sprouts, carrots, bell peppers, and onions)

- 2 tbsp olive oil
- 1 tsp lemon juice
- Salt and pepper to taste

Instructions:
1. Preheat the grill to medium-high heat.
2. Season salmon with salt, pepper, and lemon juice.
3. Grill salmon for 4-6 minutes per side or until cooked through.
4. Toss vegetables in olive oil, salt, and pepper.
5. Spread on a baking sheet and roast in the oven at 425°F (220°C) for 20-25 minutes or until tender.
6. Serve salmon with roasted vegetables.

Tips:
- Choose wild-caught salmon for lower acidity.
- Select vegetables that are easy to digest.
- Use olive oil for a healthy fat.
- Eat slowly and mindfully to alleviate GERD symptoms.

This recipe is a flavorful and nutritious option for a GERD-friendly dinner. The grilled salmon provides a lean protein source, while the roasted vegetables offer a soothing and fiber-rich complement.

2. Vegetable Stir-Fry With Tofu And Brown Rice

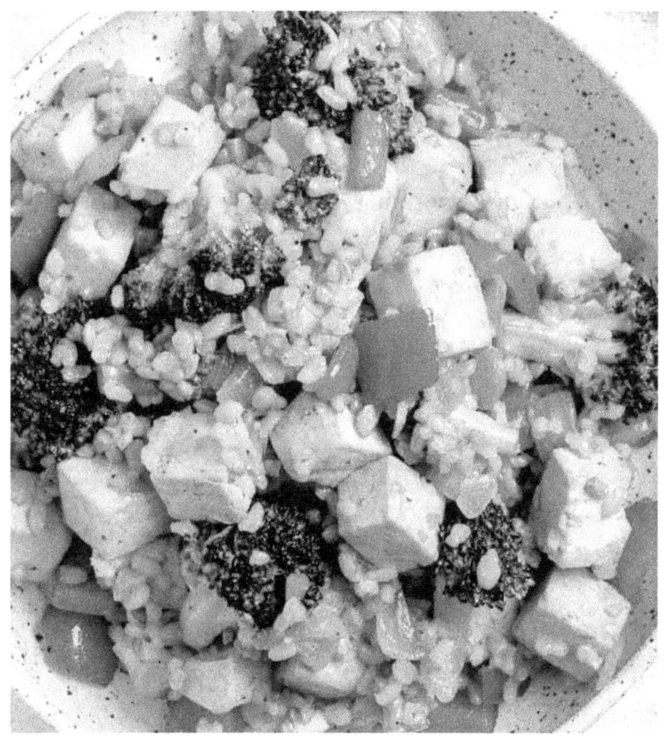

Ingredients:

- 1 cup firm tofu, cubed
- 2 cups mixed vegetables (such as broccoli, bell peppers, carrots, and mushrooms)
- 2 tablespoons olive oil
- 1 tablespoon soy sauce (low-sodium)
- 1 tablespoon honey
- 1 teaspoon grated ginger
- Salt and pepper to taste
- 1 cup cooked brown rice

Instructions:
1. Heat olive oil in a large skillet or wok over medium-high heat.
2. Add tofu and cook until golden brown.
3. Add mixed vegetables, soy sauce, honey, and ginger.
4. Stir-fry until vegetables are tender-crisp.
5. Serve over brown rice.

Tips:
- Choose low-sodium soy sauce to reduce acidity.
- Select vegetables that are easy to digest.
- Use olive oil for a healthy fat.

This recipe is a flavorful and nutritious option for a GERD-friendly dinner. The vegetable stir-fry provides a soothing and fiber-rich complement, while the tofu offers a lean protein source, and the brown rice provides a gentle and easily digestible base.

3. Lentil Soup With Whole Grain Bread

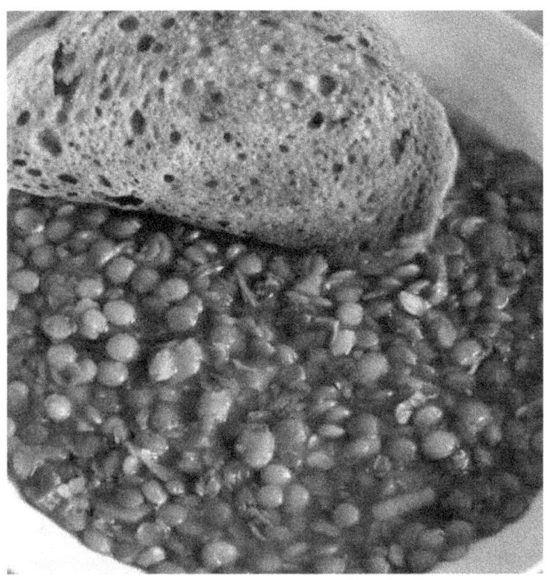

Ingredients:

- 1 cup dried green or brown lentils, rinsed and drained
- 4 cups vegetable broth (low-sodium)
- 1 onion, chopped
- 2 cloves garlic, minced
- 1 carrot, chopped
- 1 celery stalk, chopped
- 1 can diced tomatoes (low-acidity)
- 1 teaspoon dried thyme
- Salt and pepper to taste
- 2 slices whole grain bread

Instructions:

1. In a large pot, sauté onion, garlic, carrot, and celery in olive oil until tender.
2. Add lentils, vegetable broth, diced tomatoes, and thyme.
3. Bring to a boil, then reduce heat and simmer until lentils are tender.
4. Serve with whole grain bread.

Tips:
- Choose low-sodium vegetable broth to reduce acidity.
- Select low-acidity diced tomatoes.
- Use olive oil for a healthy fat.
- Eat slowly and mindfully to alleviate GERD symptoms.

This recipe is a comforting and nutritious option for a GERD-friendly dinner. The lentil soup provides a soothing and fiber-rich complement, while the whole grain bread offers a gentle and easily digestible base.

4. Grilled Chicken With Roasted Sweet Potatoes And Green Beans

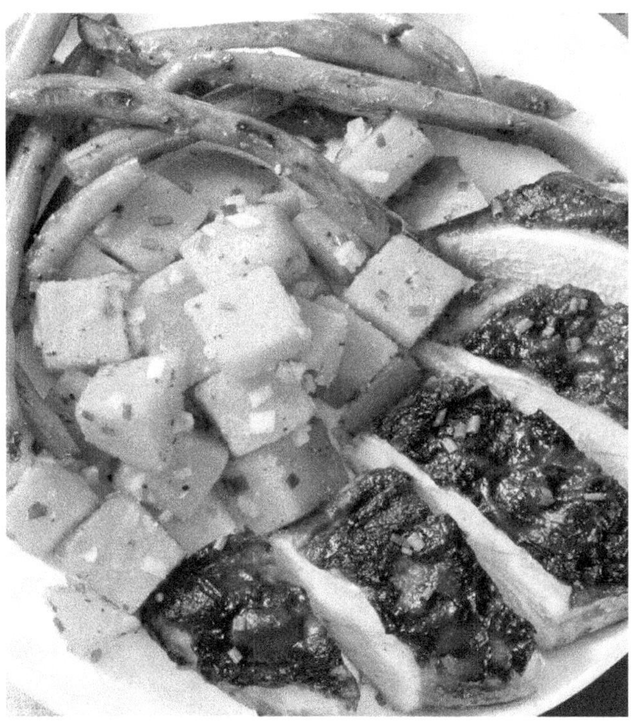

Ingredients:

- 4 oz boneless, skinless chicken breast
- 2 large sweet potatoes, peeled and cubed
- 2 cups green beans, trimmed
- 2 tbsp olive oil
- Salt and pepper to taste

Instructions:

1. Preheat the grill to medium-high heat.

2. Season chicken with salt and pepper.
3. Grill chicken for 5-6 minutes per side or until cooked through.
4. Toss sweet potatoes and green beans in olive oil, salt, and pepper.
5. Spread on a baking sheet and roast in the oven at 425°F (220°C) for 20-25 minutes or until tender.
6. Serve chicken with roasted sweet potatoes and green beans.

Tips:
- Choose lean protein like chicken breast to reduce fat and acidity.
- Select sweet potatoes for a gentle and easily digestible carbohydrate source.
- Green beans are low in acidity and easy to digest.
- Use olive oil for a healthy fat.

This recipe is a flavorful and nutritious option for a GERD-friendly dinner. The grilled chicken provides a lean protein source, while the roasted sweet potatoes and green beans offer a soothing and fiber-rich complement.

5. Quinoa And Black Bean Bowl With Roasted Vegetables

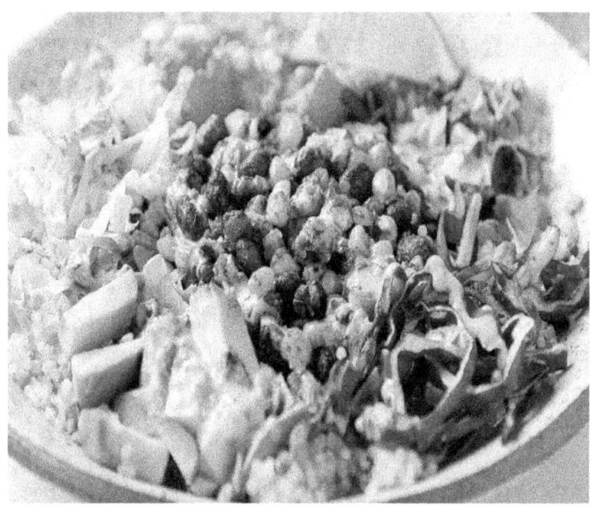

Ingredients:
- 1 cup quinoa, rinsed and drained
- 2 cups water or vegetable broth
- 1 cup cooked black beans
- 2 cups mixed roasted vegetables (such as broccoli, carrots, bell peppers, and onions)
- 2 tablespoons olive oil
- Salt and pepper to taste

Instructions:
1. Cook quinoa according to package instructions.
2. In a separate pan, heat olive oil and add black beans, salt, and pepper.
3. Stir in roasted vegetables.
4. Combine cooked quinoa and black bean mixture.

5. Serve in a bowl and enjoy.

Tips:
- Choose quinoa for a gentle and easily digestible protein source.
- Black beans are low in acidity and high in fiber.
- Select roasted vegetables that are easy to digest.
- Use olive oil for a healthy fat.

This recipe is a flavorful and nutritious option for a GERD-friendly dinner. The quinoa and black bean bowl provides a soothing and fiber-rich complement, while the roasted vegetables add a delicious and easy-to-digest element.

6. Baked Cod With Roasted Asparagus And Brown Rice

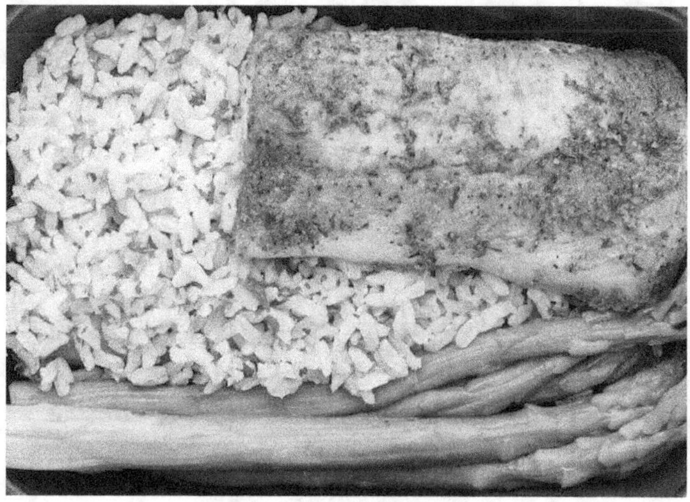

Ingredients:
- 4 oz cod filet
- 2 cups asparagus spears, trimmed
- 1 cup brown rice
- 2 tablespoons olive oil
- Salt and pepper to taste

Instructions:
1. Preheat the oven to 400°F (200°C).
2. Season cod with salt and pepper.
3. Bake in the oven for 12-15 minutes or until cooked through.
4. Toss asparagus in olive oil, salt, and pepper.
5. Spread on a baking sheet and roast in the oven for 12-15 minutes or until tender.
6. Cook brown rice according to package instructions.
7. Serve cod with roasted asparagus and brown rice.

Tips:
- Choose cod for a lean protein source that's low in acidity.
- Asparagus is a low-acidity vegetable that's easy to digest.
- Brown rice is a gentle and easily digestible carbohydrate source.
- Use olive oil for a healthy fat.

This recipe is a flavorful and nutritious option for a GERD-friendly dinner. The baked cod provides a lean protein source, while the roasted asparagus and brown rice offer a soothing and fiber-rich complement.

7. Vegetable Curry With Brown Rice And Whole Grain Naan

Ingredients:
- 2 cups mixed vegetables (such as bell peppers, carrots, potatoes, and green beans)
- 2 tablespoons curry powder
- 1 teaspoon turmeric
- 1 teaspoon cumin
- 1 can coconut milk (low-fat)
- 1 cup brown rice
- 2 whole grain naan bread
- 2 tablespoons olive oil
- Salt and pepper to taste

Instructions:
1. Heat olive oil in a large pan over medium heat.
2. Add onions, ginger, and garlic for 2-3 minutes.
3. Add mixed vegetables, curry powder, turmeric, and cumin. Cook for 5 minutes.
4. Stir in coconut milk and bring to a simmer.
5. Cook brown rice according to package instructions.
6. Warm whole grain naan bread in the oven.
7. Serve vegetable curry over brown rice with naan bread on the side.

Tips:
- Choose low-fat coconut milk to reduce acidity.
- Select whole grain naan bread for a gentle and easily digestible carbohydrate source.
- Brown rice is a soothing and fiber-rich complement.
- Use olive oil for a healthy fat.

This recipe is a flavorful and nutritious option for a GERD-friendly dinner. The vegetable curry provides a soothing and fiber-rich complement, while the brown rice and whole grain naan offer a gentle and easily digestible base.

8. Grilled Turkey Burger On Whole Grain Bread With Roasted Vegetables

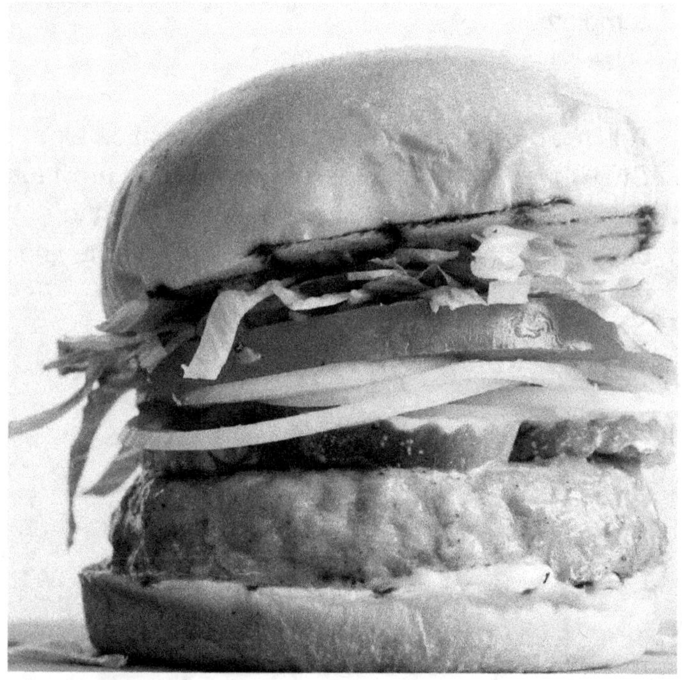

Ingredients:
- 4 oz ground turkey breast
- 1 whole grain bread bun
- 2 cups mixed roasted vegetables (such as lettuce, tomato, bell peppers, and onions)
- 2 tablespoons olive oil
- Salt and pepper to taste

Instructions:

1. Preheat the grill to medium-high heat.
2. Form ground turkey into a patty.
3. Grill for 5-6 minutes per side or until cooked through.
4. Toast whole grain bread bun.
5. Top with turkey patty, roasted vegetables, and olive oil.
6. Serve immediately.

Tips:
- Choose lean ground turkey breast to reduce fat and acidity.
- Select whole grain bread for a gentle and easily digestible carbohydrate source.
- Roasted vegetables are low in acidity and easy to digest.
- Use olive oil for a healthy fat.

This recipe is a flavorful and nutritious option for a GERD-friendly dinner. The grilled turkey burger provides a lean protein source, while the whole grain bread and roasted vegetables offer a soothing and fiber-rich complement.

9. Slow Cooker Beef Stew With Whole Grain Crackers

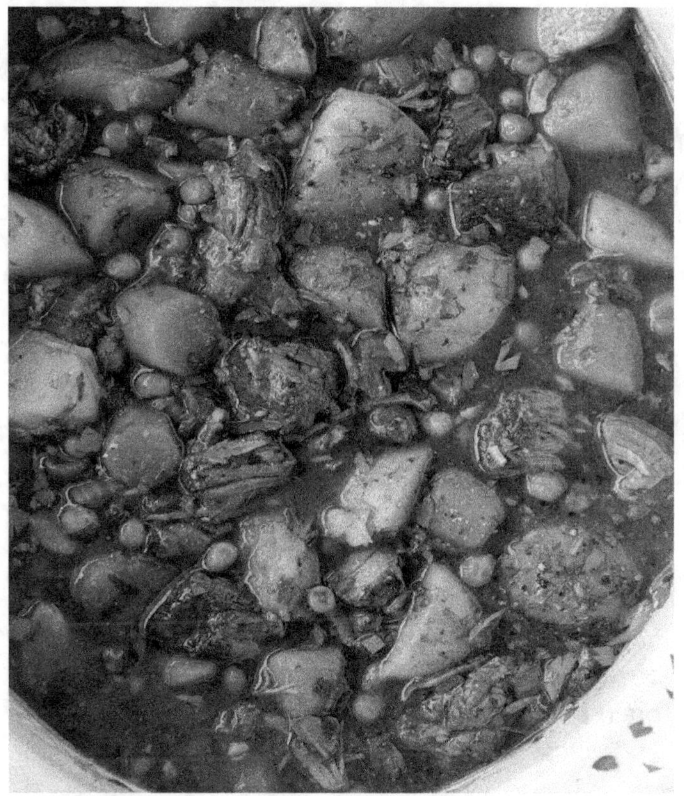

Ingredients:
- 2 pounds beef stew meat (lean cut)
- 2 cups mixed vegetables (such as carrots, potatoes, and green beans)
- 2 cups beef broth (low-sodium)
- 1 teaspoon dried thyme
- 1/2 teaspoon dried rosemary
- 1 bay leaf

- 2 whole grain crackers

Instructions:
1. Add beef, vegetables, beef broth, thyme, rosemary, and bay leaf to the slow cooker.
2. Cook on low for 8-10 hours or high for 4-6 hours.
3. Serve with whole grain crackers.

Tips:
- Choose lean beef stew meat to reduce fat and acidity.
- Select low-sodium beef broth to reduce acidity.
- Whole grain crackers are a gentle and easily digestible carbohydrate source.
- Eat slowly and mindfully to alleviate GERD symptoms.

This recipe is a comforting and nutritious option for a GERD-friendly dinner. The slow cooker beef stew provides a soothing and fiber-rich complement, while the whole grain crackers offer a gentle and easily digestible base.

10. Roasted Vegetables And Bean Tacos With Whole Grain Tortillas

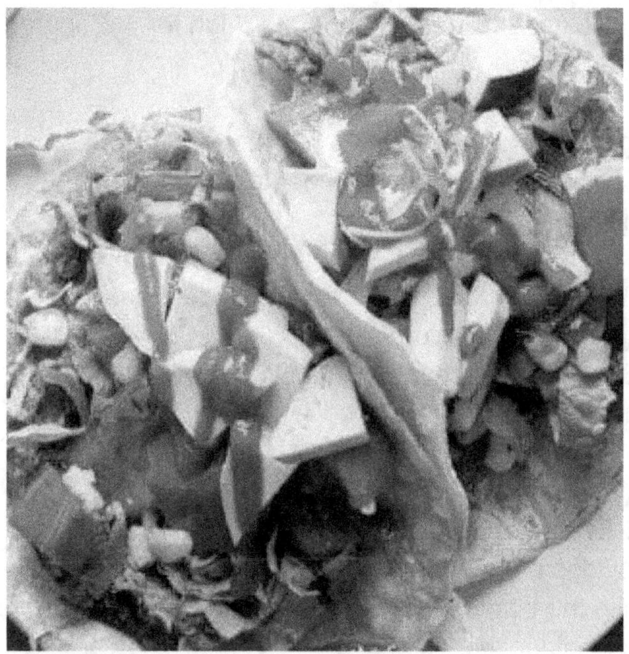

Ingredients:

- 2 cups mixed roasted vegetables (such as bell peppers, zucchini, and onions)
- 1 cup cooked black beans
- 2 whole grain tortillas
- 2 tablespoons olive oil
- 1 tablespoon lime juice
- Salt and pepper to taste
- Optional: avocado, salsa, and shredded lettuce

Instructions:
1. Roast vegetables in olive oil until tender.
2. Warm whole grain tortillas in the oven.
3. Fill tortillas with roasted vegetables, black beans, and desired toppings.
4. Serve immediately.

Tips:
- Choose whole grain tortillas for a gentle and easily digestible carbohydrate source.
- Black beans are low in acidity and high in fiber.
- Roasted vegetables are easy to digest and low in acidity.
- Use olive oil for a healthy fat.

This recipe is a flavorful and nutritious option for a GERD-friendly dinner. The roasted vegetables and black beans provide a soothing and fiber-rich complement, while the whole grain tortillas offer a gentle and easily digestible base.

11. Grilled Shrimp With Roasted Brussels Sprouts And Quinoa

Ingredients:
- 12 large shrimp, peeled and deveined
- 2 cups Brussels sprouts, trimmed and halved
- 1 cup quinoa, rinsed and drained
- 2 tablespoons olive oil
- Salt and pepper to taste

Instructions:
1. Preheat the grill to medium-high heat.
2. Grill shrimp for 2-3 minutes per side or until cooked through.
3. Toss Brussels sprouts in olive oil, salt, and pepper.
4. Roast in the oven at 400°F (200°C) for 20-25 minutes or until tender.
5. Cook quinoa according to package instructions.
6. Serve shrimp with roasted Brussels sprouts and quinoa.

Tips:
- Choose lean protein like shrimp to reduce fat and acidity.
- Brussels sprouts are low in acidity and high in fiber.
- Quinoa is a gentle and easily digestible carbohydrate source.
- Use olive oil for a healthy fat.

This recipe is a flavorful and nutritious option for a GERD-friendly dinner. The grilled shrimp provides a lean protein source, while the roasted Brussels sprouts and quinoa offer a soothing and fiber-rich complement.

12. Vegetable And Lentil Curry With Brown Rice

Ingredients:

- 1 cup brown rice
- 2 cups water or vegetable broth
- 1 cup red or green lentils, rinsed and drained
- 2 cups mixed vegetables (such as carrots, potatoes, and green beans)
- 2 tablespoons curry powder
- 1 teaspoon turmeric
- 1 teaspoon cumin
- 1 can coconut milk (low-fat)
- 2 tablespoons olive oil
- Salt and pepper to taste

Instructions:
1. Cook brown rice according to package instructions.
2. In a large pot, sauté onions, ginger, and garlic in olive oil.
3. Add lentils, vegetables, curry powder, turmeric, and cumin.
4. Stir in coconut milk and water or broth.
5. Bring to a simmer and cook until lentils are tender.
6. Serve curry over brown rice.

Tips:
- Choose low-fat coconut milk to reduce acidity.
- Lentils are low in acidity and high in fiber.
- Brown rice is a gentle and easily digestible carbohydrate source.
- Use olive oil for a healthy fat.

This recipe is a flavorful and nutritious option for a GERD-friendly dinner. The vegetable and lentil curry provides a soothing and fiber-rich complement, while the brown rice offers a gentle and easily digestible base.

13. Baked Chicken With Roasted Carrots And Brown Rice

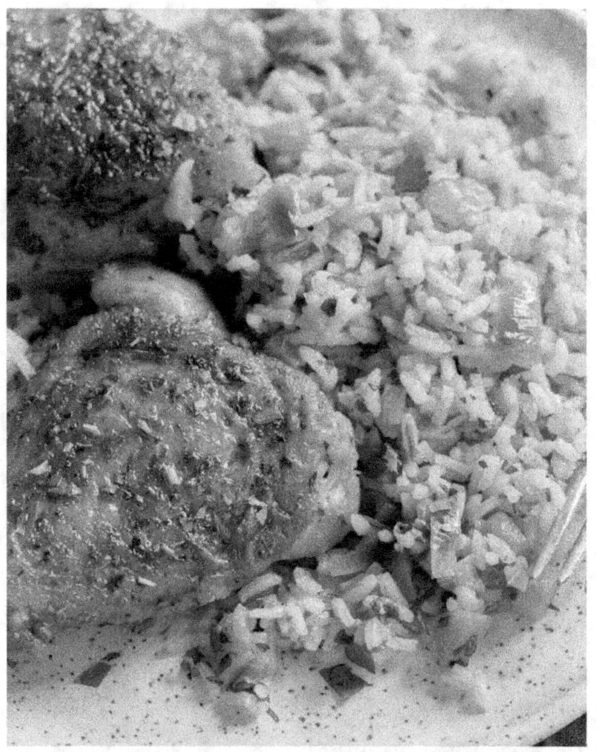

Ingredients:
- 4 oz boneless, skinless chicken breast

- 2 cups carrots, peeled and chopped
- 1 cup brown rice
- 2 tablespoons olive oil
- Salt and pepper to taste

Instructions:
1. Preheat the oven to 400°F (200°C).
2. Season chicken with salt and pepper.
3. Bake in the oven for 20-25 minutes or until cooked through.
4. Toss carrots in olive oil, salt, and pepper.
5. Roast in the oven for 20-25 minutes or until tender.
6. Cook brown rice according to package instructions.
7. Serve chicken with roasted carrots and brown rice.

Tips:
- Choose lean protein like chicken breast to reduce fat and acidity.
- Carrots are low in acidity and easy to digest.
- Brown rice is a gentle and easily digestible carbohydrate source.
- Use olive oil for a healthy fat.

This recipe is a flavorful and nutritious option for a GERD-friendly dinner. The baked chicken provides a lean protein source, while the roasted carrots and brown rice offer a soothing and fiber-rich complement.

14. Grilled Pork Chop With Roasted Bell Peppers And Sweet Potatoes

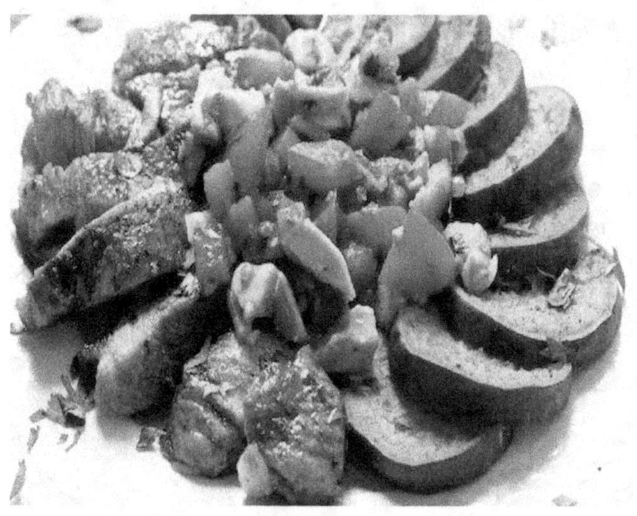

Ingredients:
- 4 oz pork chop
- 2 cups mixed bell peppers, seeded and sliced
- 2 large sweet potatoes, peeled and cubed
- 2 tablespoons olive oil
- Salt and pepper to taste

Instructions:
1. Preheat the grill to medium-high heat.
2. Grill pork chop for 5-6 minutes per side or until cooked through.
3. Toss bell peppers and sweet potatoes in olive oil, salt, and pepper.

4. Roast in the oven at 425°F (220°C) for 25-30 minutes or until tender.
5. Serve pork chop with roasted bell peppers and sweet potatoes.

Tips:
- Choose lean protein like pork chop to reduce fat and acidity.
- Bell peppers are low in acidity and easy to digest.
- Sweet potatoes are a gentle and easily digestible carbohydrate source.
- Use olive oil for a healthy fat.

This recipe is a flavorful and nutritious option for a GERD-friendly dinner. The grilled pork chop provides a lean protein source, while the roasted bell peppers and sweet potatoes offer a soothing and fiber-rich complement.

15. Grilled Chicken Breast With Roasted Asparagus And Quinoa

Ingredients:
- 4 oz chicken breast
- 2 cups asparagus spears, trimmed
- 1 cup quinoa, rinsed and drained
- 2 tablespoons olive oil
- Salt and pepper to taste

Instructions:
1. Preheat the grill to medium-high heat.

2. Grill chicken breast for 5-6 minutes per side or until cooked through.
3. Toss asparagus in olive oil, salt, and pepper.
4. Roast in the oven at 425°F (220°C) for 12-15 minutes or until tender.
5. Cook quinoa according to package instructions.
6. Serve chicken breast with roasted asparagus and quinoa.

Tips:
- Choose lean protein like chicken breast to reduce fat and acidity.
- Asparagus is low in acidity and easy to digest.
- Quinoa is a gentle and easily digestible carbohydrate source.
- Use olive oil for a healthy fat.

This recipe is a flavorful and nutritious option for a GERD-friendly dinner. The grilled chicken breast provides a lean protein source, while the roasted asparagus and quinoa offer a soothing and fiber-rich complement.

16. Black Beans And Corn Chili With Whole Grain Crackers

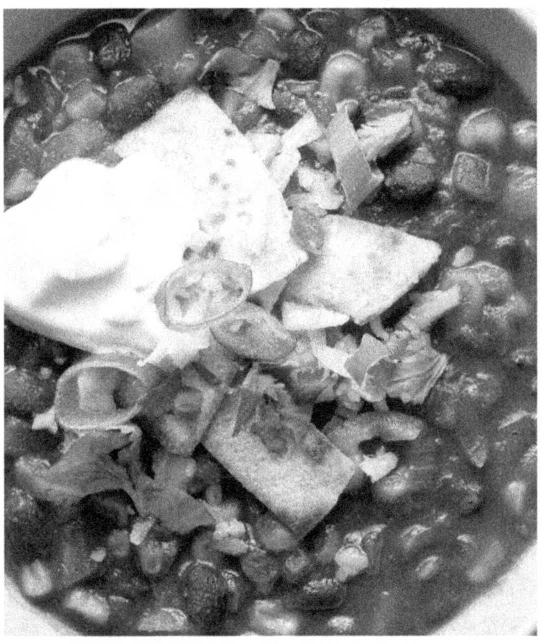

Ingredients:
- 1 cup dried black beans, cooked
- 1 cup frozen corn kernels
- 1 can diced tomatoes
- 1 onion, diced
- 2 cloves garlic, minced
- 1 teaspoon cumin
- 1 teaspoon chili powder
- Salt and pepper to taste
- 6 whole grain crackers

Instructions:

1. In a pot, sauté onion and garlic until softened.
2. Add cumin and chili powder for 1 minute.
3. Stir in black beans, corn, and diced tomatoes.
4. Simmer for 20-25 minutes or until heated through.
5. Serve with whole grain crackers.

Tips:
- Black beans are low in acidity and high in fiber.
- Corn is easy to digest and low in acidity.
- Whole grain crackers are a gentle and easily digestible carbohydrate source.
- Avoid adding hot peppers or spicy seasonings to reduce acidity.

This recipe is a flavorful and nutritious option for a GERD-friendly dinner. The black beans and corn chili provides a soothing and fiber-rich complement, while the whole grain crackers offer a gentle and easily digestible base.

17. Grilled Steak With Roasted Broccoli And Quinoa

Ingredients:
- 6 oz steak (choose a lean cut like sirloin or tenderloin)
- 2 cups broccoli florets
- 1 cup quinoa, rinsed and drained
- 2 tablespoons olive oil
- Salt and pepper to taste

Instructions:
1. Preheat the grill to medium-high heat.
2. Grill steak for 5-7 minutes per side or until cooked to desired doneness.
3. Toss broccoli in olive oil, salt, and pepper.
4. Roast in the oven at 425°F (220°C) for 15-20 minutes or until tender.
5. Cook quinoa according to package instructions.
6. Serve steak with roasted broccoli and quinoa.

Tips:
- Choose lean protein like steak to reduce fat and acidity.
- Broccoli is low in acidity and easy to digest.
- Quinoa is a gentle and easily digestible carbohydrate source.
- Use olive oil for a healthy fat.

This recipe is a flavorful and nutritious option for a GERD-friendly dinner. The grilled steak provides a lean protein source, while the roasted broccoli and quinoa offer a soothing and fiber-rich complement.

18. Roasted Vegetables And Hummus Wrap With WholeGrain Wrap

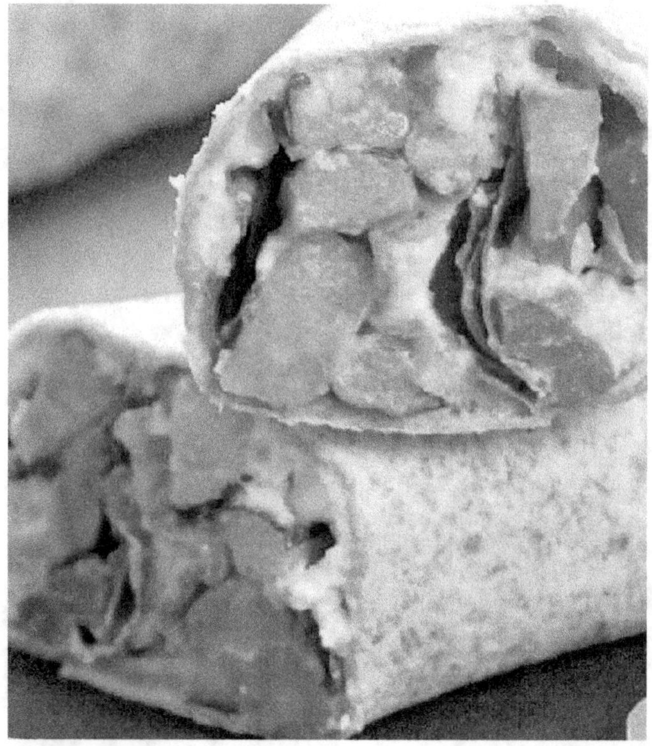

Ingredients:
- 1 whole grain wrap
- 1/2 cup hummus
- 2 cups mixed roasted vegetables (such as bell peppers, zucchini, eggplant, and red onion)
- 2 tablespoons olive oil
- Salt and pepper to taste

Instructions:

1. Preheat the oven to 425°F (220°C).
2. Toss vegetables in olive oil, salt, and pepper.
3. Roast in the oven for 25-30 minutes or until tender.
4. Spread hummus on the whole grain wrap.
5. Add roasted vegetables and wrap up.

Tips:

- Choose whole grain wrap for a gentle and easily digestible carbohydrate source.
- Hummus is low in acidity and high in fiber.
- Roasted vegetables are easy to digest and low in acidity.
- Use olive oil for a healthy fat.

This recipe is a flavorful and nutritious option for a GERD-friendly dinner. The roasted vegetables and hummus provide a soothing and fiber-rich complement, while the whole grain wrap offers a gentle and easily digestible base.

19. Baked Cod With Roasted Cauliflower And Brown Rice

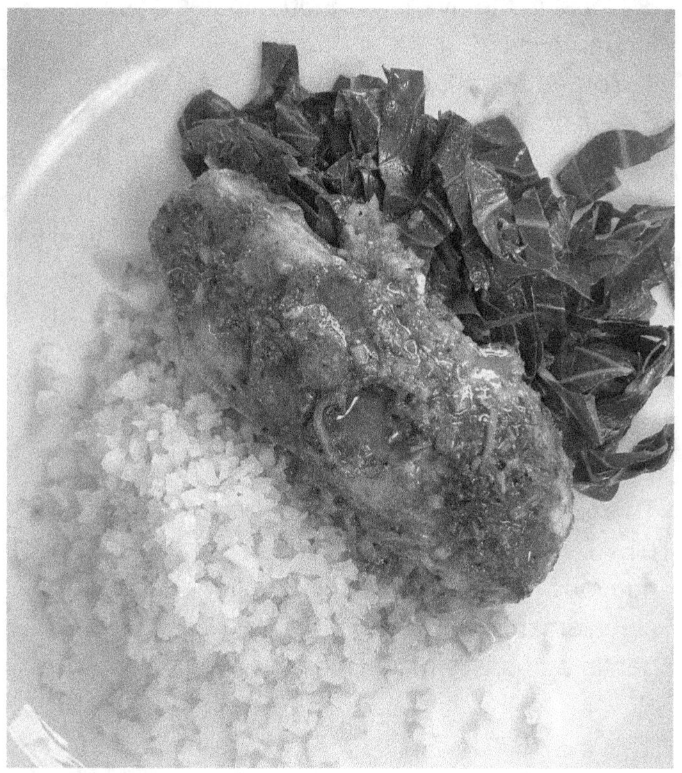

Ingredients:

- 6 oz cod filet
- 2 cups cauliflower florets
- 1 cup brown rice
- 2 tablespoons olive oil
- Salt and pepper to taste

Instructions:

1. Preheat the oven to 400°F (200°C).

2. Season cod with salt and pepper.
3. Bake in the oven for 12-15 minutes or until cooked through.
4. Toss cauliflower in olive oil, salt, and pepper.
5. Roast in the oven for 20-25 minutes or until tender.
6. Cook brown rice according to package instructions.
7. Serve cod with roasted cauliflower and brown rice.

Tips:
- Choose lean protein like cod to reduce fat and acidity.
- Cauliflower is low in acidity and easy to digest.
- Brown rice is a gentle and easily digestible carbohydrate source.
- Use olive oil for a healthy fat.
- Eat slowly and mindfully to alleviate GERD symptoms.

This recipe is a flavorful and nutritious option for a GERD-friendly dinner. The baked cod provides a lean protein source, while the roasted cauliflower and brown rice offer a soothing and fiber-rich complement.

20. Vegetable And Bean Chili With Whole Grain CornBread

Ingredients:

- 1 cup dried beans (such as kidney or black beans)
- 2 cups mixed vegetables (such as bell peppers, onions, and tomatoes)
- 2 cups vegetable broth
- 1 teaspoon chili powder
- 1 teaspoon cumin
- 1 whole grain cornbread mix
- 1 cup water

Instructions:
1. Cook beans and vegetables in vegetable broth with chili powder and cumin.
2. Simmer for 20-25 minutes or until the beans are tender.
3. Prepare whole grain cornbread mix according to package instructions.
4. Bake in the oven for 20-25 minutes or until a toothpick comes out clean.
5. Serve chili with whole grain cornbread.

Tips:
- Choose low-acidity vegetables like bell peppers and onions.
- Beans are low in acidity and high in fiber.
- Whole grain cornbread is a gentle and easily digestible carbohydrate source.
- Avoid adding hot peppers or spicy seasonings to reduce acidity.

This recipe is a flavorful and nutritious option for a GERD-friendly dinner. The vegetable and bean chili provides a soothing and fiber-rich complement, while the whole grain cornbread offers a gentle and easily digestible base.

Chapter Three

Soups And Stews

1. Vegetable Broth With Lean Beef

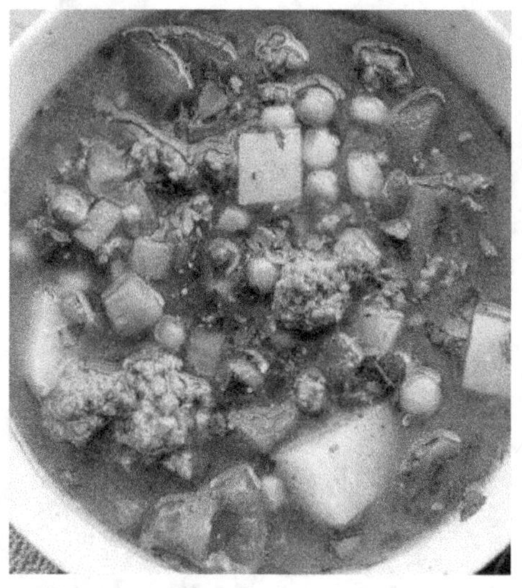

Ingredients:

- 1 pound lean beef (such as sirloin or round), sliced into thin strips
- 4 cups vegetable broth (low-sodium)
- 1 large onion, chopped
- 2 cloves garlic, minced
- 2 carrots, peeled and chopped
- 2 celery stalks, chopped
- 2 potatoes, peeled and chopped

- 1 teaspoon dried thyme
- 1/2 teaspoon dried basil
- Salt and pepper, to taste

Instructions:

1. In a large pot, combine beef, vegetable broth, onion, garlic, carrots, celery, potatoes, thyme, and basil.
2. Bring to a boil, then reduce heat and simmer for 1 1/2 hours or until beef is tender.
3. Season with salt and pepper to taste.
4. Serve hot, garnished with fresh herbs (optional).

Tips:
- Use lean beef to reduce fat content.
- Choose low-sodium vegetable broth to reduce acidity.
- Avoid adding tomatoes or citrus, which can trigger GERD symptoms.
- Cook slowly and gently to prevent acid reflux.

This recipe is gentle on the stomach and esophagus, making it suitable for those with GERD. The lean beef provides protein, while the vegetables add fiber and nutrients.

2. Chicken And Rice Soup With Low-Fat Chicken

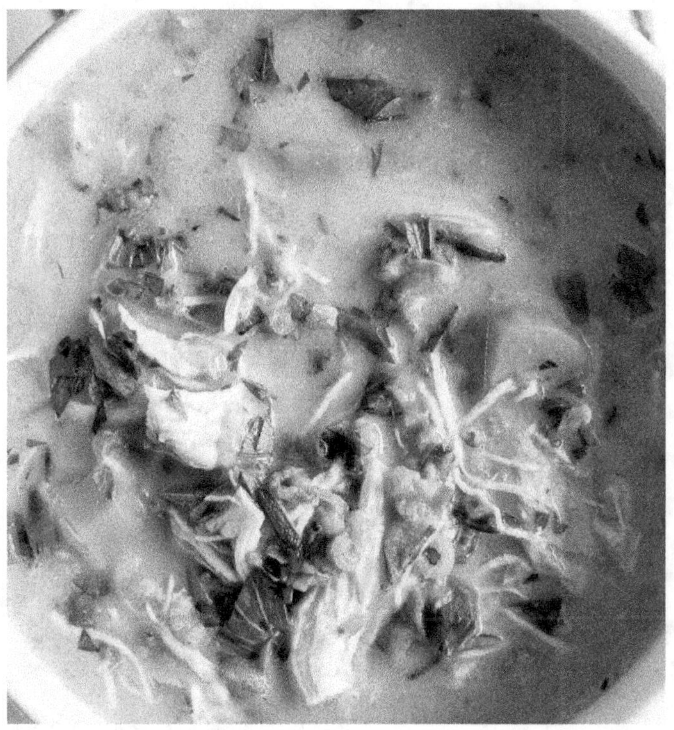

Ingredients:
- 1 pound boneless, skinless chicken breast or tenderloins, cut into small pieces
- 2 cups low-sodium chicken broth
- 1 cup uncooked white or brown rice
- 1 large onion, chopped
- 2 cloves garlic, minced
- 2 carrots, peeled and chopped
- 2 celery stalks, chopped
- 1 teaspoon dried thyme

- Salt and pepper, to taste

Instructions:
1. In a large pot, sauté the chicken, onion, garlic, carrots, and celery in a little water until the chicken is browned and the vegetables are tender.
2. Add the chicken broth, rice, thyme, salt, and pepper.
3. Bring to a boil, then reduce heat and simmer for 20-25 minutes or until the rice is cooked and the liquid has been absorbed.
4. Serve hot, garnished with fresh herbs (optional).

Tips:
- Use low-fat chicken breast or tenderloins to reduce fat content.
- Choose low-sodium chicken broth to reduce acidity.
- Avoid adding tomatoes or citrus, which can trigger GERD symptoms.
- Cook slowly and gently to prevent acid reflux.

This recipe is gentle on the stomach and esophagus. The low-fat chicken provides protein, while the rice and vegetables add fiber and nutrients.

3. Chicken And Vegetable Soup With Whole Grain Pasta

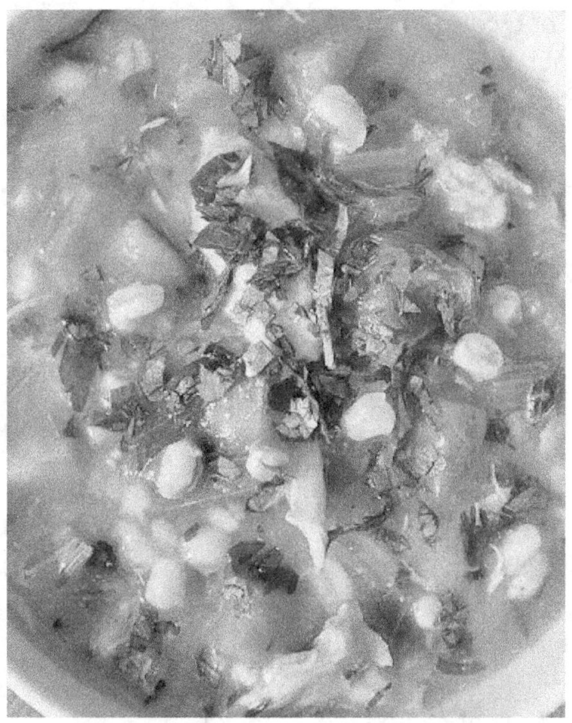

Ingredients:
- 1 pound boneless, skinless chicken breast or tenderloins, cut into small pieces
- 2 cups low-sodium chicken broth
- 1 cup whole grain pasta (such as brown rice pasta or quinoa pasta)
- 1 large onion, chopped
- 2 cloves garlic, minced
- 2 carrots, peeled and chopped

- 2 celery stalks, chopped
- 1 cup mixed vegetables (such as green beans, zucchini, and bell peppers)
- 1 teaspoon dried basil
- Salt and pepper, to taste

Instructions:
1. In a large pot, sauté the chicken, onion, garlic, carrots, and celery in a little water until the chicken is browned and the vegetables are tender.
2. Add the chicken broth, whole grain pasta, mixed vegetables, and basil.
3. Bring to a boil, then reduce heat and simmer for 20-25 minutes or until the pasta is al dente and the vegetables are tender.
4. Season with salt and pepper to taste.
5. Serve hot, garnished with fresh herbs (optional).

Tips:
- Use low-fat chicken breast or tenderloins to reduce fat content.
- Choose low-sodium chicken broth to reduce acidity.
- Select whole grain pasta to increase fiber content.
- Avoid adding tomatoes or citrus, which can trigger GERD symptoms.
- Cook slowly and gently to prevent acid reflux.

The whole grain pasta adds fiber, while the vegetables provide essential nutrients.

4. Vegetable Stew With Lean Pork And Quinoa

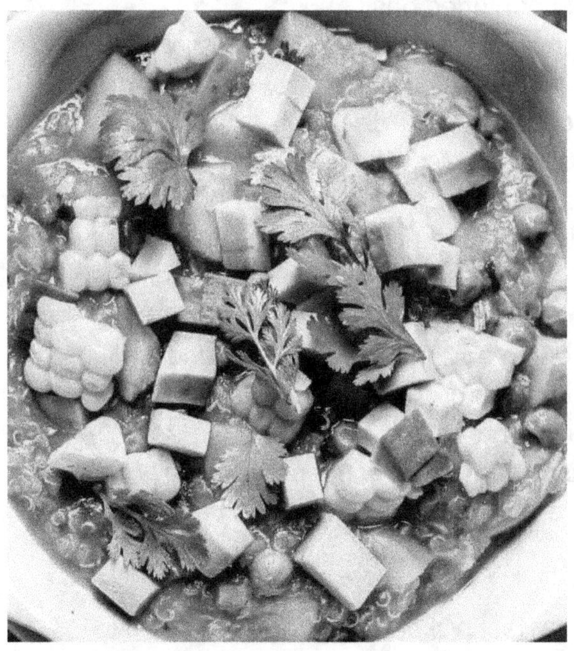

Ingredients:

- 1 pound lean pork tenderloin, cut into small pieces
- 2 cups mixed vegetables (such as carrots, zucchini, green beans, and bell peppers)
- 1 cup quinoa
- 2 cups low-sodium vegetable broth
- 1 large onion, chopped
- 2 cloves garlic, minced
- 1 teaspoon dried thyme
- Salt and pepper, to taste

Instructions:

1. In a large pot, sauté the pork, onion, and garlic in a little water until the pork is browned.
2. Add the mixed vegetables, quinoa, vegetable broth, and thyme.
3. Bring to a boil, then reduce heat and simmer for 25-30 minutes or until the quinoa is tender and the vegetables are cooked.
4. Season with salt and pepper to taste.
5. Serve hot, garnished with fresh herbs (optional).

Tips:
- Use lean pork tenderloin to reduce fat content.
- Choose low-sodium vegetable broth to reduce acidity.
- Select quinoa as a whole grain to increase fiber content.
- Avoid adding tomatoes or citrus, which can trigger GERD symptoms.
- Cook slowly and gently to prevent acid reflux.

The lean pork provides protein, while the quinoa and vegetables add fiber and essential nutrients.

5. Butternut Squash Soup With Low-Fat Coconut Milk

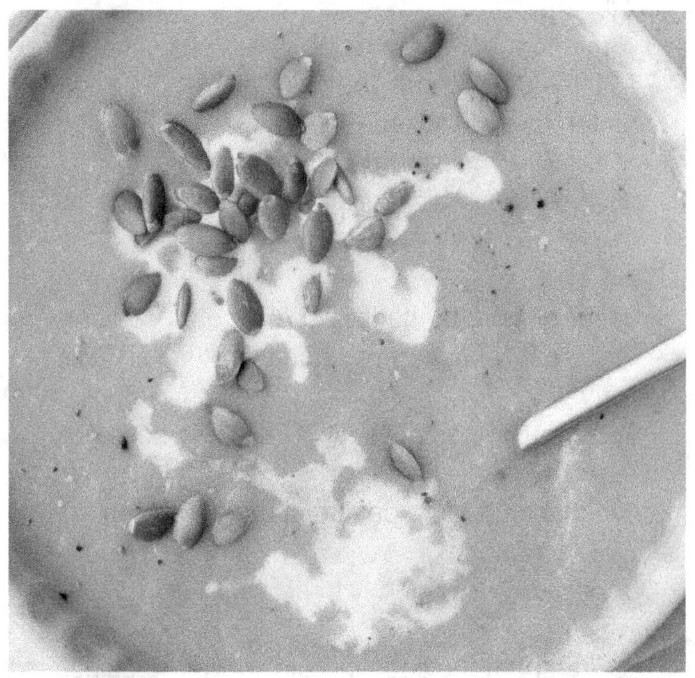

Ingredients:

- 1 medium butternut squash (about 2 pounds)
- 2 cups low-sodium vegetable broth
- 1/2 cup low-fat coconut milk
- 1 large onion, chopped
- 2 cloves garlic, minced
- 1 teaspoon ground cumin
- 1 teaspoon ground coriander
- Salt and pepper, to taste

Instructions:

1. Preheat the oven to 400°F (200°C).
2. Cut the butternut squash in half lengthwise and scoop out the seeds.
3. Place the squash on a baking sheet, cut side up, and roast for 45 minutes or until tender.
4. Scoop the flesh into a pot and add the vegetable broth, onion, garlic, cumin, coriander, salt, and pepper.
5. Bring to a boil, then reduce heat and simmer for 15-20 minutes or until the soup is smooth.
6. Stir in the low-fat coconut milk and adjust seasoning as needed.
7. Serve hot, garnished with fresh herbs (optional).

Tips:
- Use low-sodium vegetable broth to reduce acidity.
- Choose low-fat coconut milk to reduce fat content.
- Avoid adding spicy or acidic ingredients, which can trigger GERD symptoms.
- Cook slowly and gently to prevent acid reflux.

The butternut squash provides fiber and essential nutrients, while the low-fat coconut milk adds creaminess without excess fat.

6. Chicken And Vegetable Stew With Brown Rice

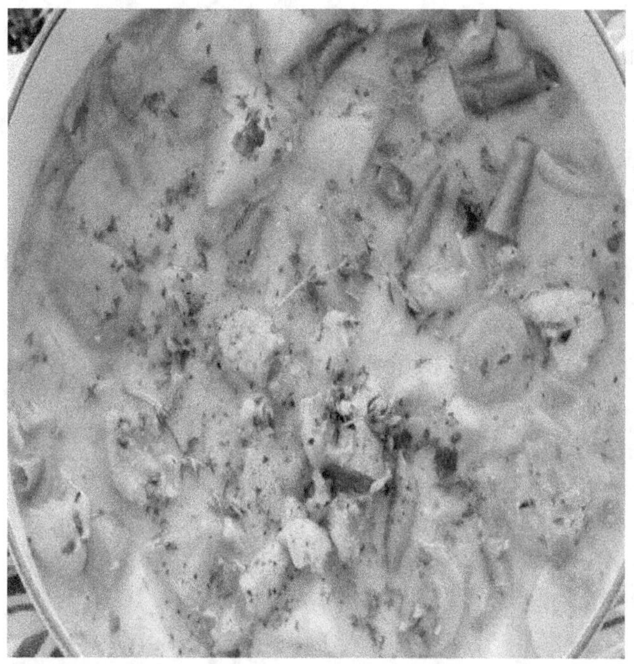

Ingredients:
- 1 pound boneless, skinless chicken breast or thighs, cut into small pieces
- 2 cups mixed vegetables (such as carrots, potatoes, green beans, and peas)
- 2 cups low-sodium chicken broth
- 1 cup brown rice
- 1 large onion, chopped
- 2 cloves garlic, minced
- 1 teaspoon dried thyme
- Salt and pepper, to taste

Instructions:
1. In a large pot, sauté the chicken, onion, and garlic in a little water until the chicken is browned.
2. Add the mixed vegetables, chicken broth, brown rice, and thyme.
3. Bring to a boil, then reduce heat and simmer for 25-30 minutes or until the rice is tender and the vegetables are cooked.
4. Season with salt and pepper to taste.
5. Serve hot, garnished with fresh herbs (optional).

Tips:
- Use lean chicken breast or thighs to reduce fat content.
- Choose low-sodium chicken broth to reduce acidity.
- Select brown rice as a whole grain to increase fiber content.
- Avoid adding tomatoes or citrus, which can trigger GERD symptoms.
- Cook slowly and gently to prevent acid reflux.

The lean chicken provides protein, while the brown rice and vegetables add fiber and essential nutrients.

7. Lentil And Vegetable Stew With Whole Grain Crackers

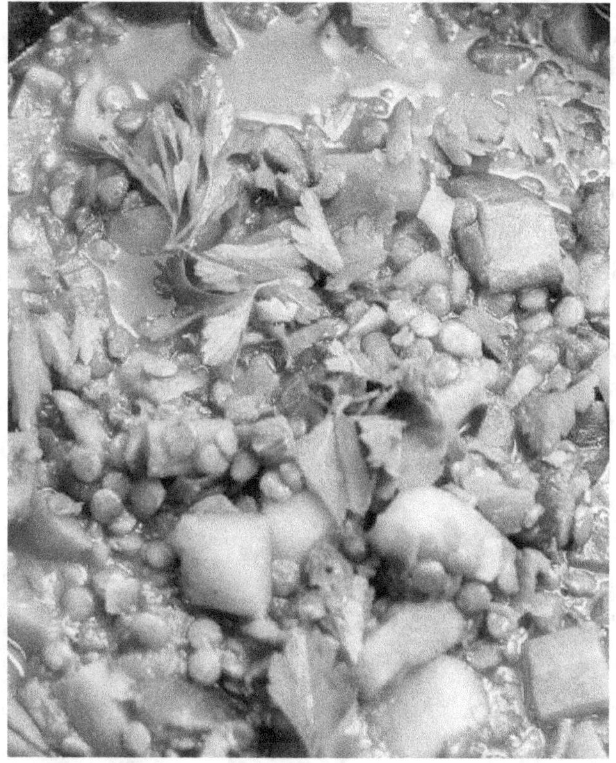

Ingredients:
- 1 cup dried green or brown lentils, rinsed and drained
- 2 cups mixed vegetables (such as carrots, potatoes, zucchini, and spinach)
- 2 cups low-sodium vegetable broth
- 1 large onion, chopped
- 2 cloves garlic, minced
- 1 teaspoon dried thyme

- 1/2 teaspoon ground cumin
- Salt and pepper, to taste
- 6-8 whole grain crackers (such as oat or rice crackers)

Instructions:
1. In a large pot, sauté the onion and garlic in a little water until softened.
2. Add the lentils, mixed vegetables, vegetable broth, thyme, and cumin.
3. Bring to a boil, then reduce heat and simmer for 25-30 minutes or until the lentils are tender.
4. Season with salt and pepper to taste.
5. Serve with whole grain crackers on the side.

Tips:
- Use low-sodium vegetable broth to reduce acidity.
- Choose whole grain crackers to increase fiber content.
- Avoid adding spicy or acidic ingredients, which can trigger GERD symptoms.
- Cook slowly and gently to prevent acid reflux.

The lentils provide protein and fiber, while the whole grain crackers add additional fiber and nutrients.

8. Vegetable And Bean Soup With Low-Fat Ground Turkey

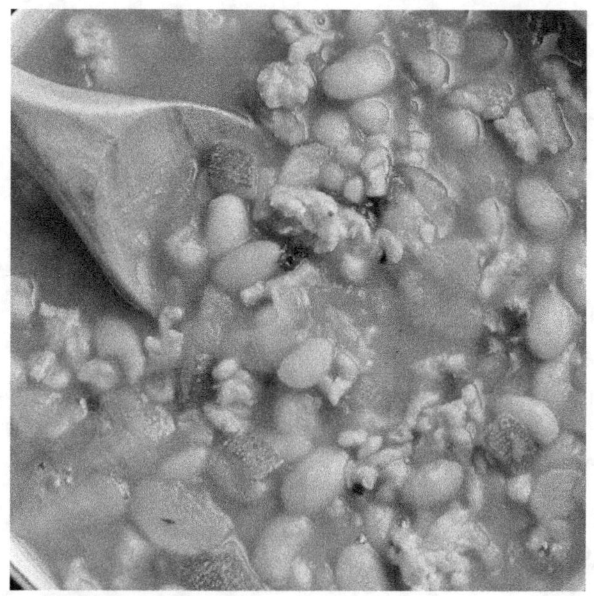

Ingredients:

- 1 pound low-fat ground turkey
- 2 cups mixed vegetables (such as carrots, zucchini, bell peppers, and tomatoes)
- 1 cup cooked kidney beans
- 2 cups low-sodium vegetable broth
- 1 large onion, chopped
- 2 cloves garlic, minced
- 1 teaspoon dried oregano
- Salt and pepper, to taste

Instructions:

1. In a large pot, cook the ground turkey over medium heat until browned, breaking it up into small pieces.
2. Add the mixed vegetables, kidney beans, vegetable broth, onion, garlic, and oregano.
3. Bring to a boil, then reduce heat and simmer for 20-25 minutes or until the vegetables are tender.
4. Season with salt and pepper to taste.
5. Serve hot, garnished with fresh herbs (optional).

Tips:
- Use low-fat ground turkey to reduce fat content.
- Choose low-sodium vegetable broth to reduce acidity.
- Avoid adding spicy or acidic ingredients, which can trigger GERD symptoms.
- Cook slowly and gently to prevent acid reflux.

The low-fat ground turkey provides protein, while the vegetables and beans add fiber and essential nutrients.

9. Chicken And Mushroom Stew With Whole Grain Noodles

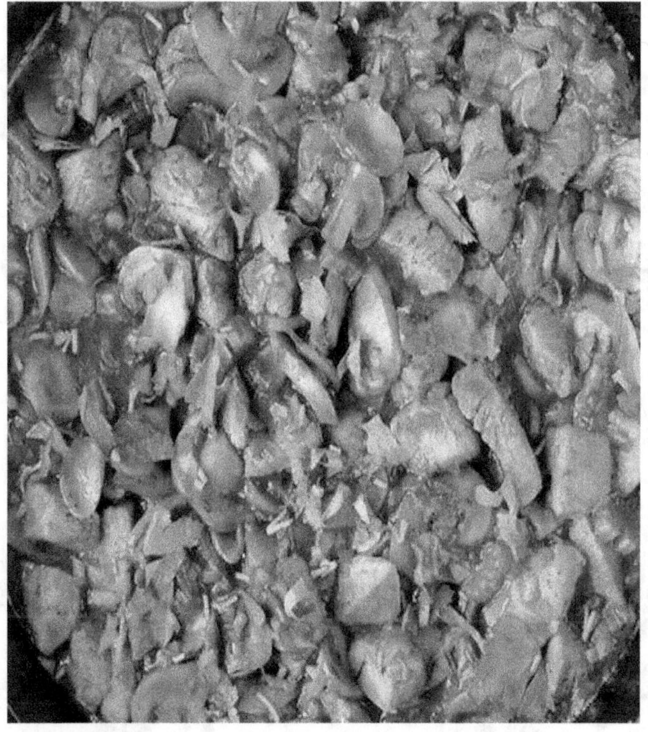

Ingredients:
- 1 pound boneless, skinless chicken breast or thighs, cut into small pieces
- 2 cups mixed mushrooms (such as button, cremini, and shiitake)
- 2 cups low-sodium chicken broth
- 1 cup whole grain noodles (such as brown rice noodles or quinoa noodles)
- 1 large onion, chopped
- 2 cloves garlic, minced

- 1 teaspoon dried thyme
- Salt and pepper, to taste

Instructions:
1. In a large pot, sauté the chicken, onion, and garlic in a little water until the chicken is browned.
2. Add the mixed mushrooms, chicken broth, whole grain noodles, and thyme.
3. Bring to a boil, then reduce heat and simmer for 20-25 minutes or until the noodles are tender and the chicken is cooked.
4. Season with salt and pepper to taste.
5. Serve hot, garnished with fresh herbs (optional).

Tips:
- Use lean chicken breast or thighs to reduce fat content.
- Choose low-sodium chicken broth to reduce acidity.
- Select whole grain noodles to increase fiber content.
- Avoid adding spicy or acidic ingredients, which can trigger GERD symptoms.
- Cook slowly and gently to prevent acid reflux.

This recipe is gentle on the stomach and esophagus, making it suitable for those with GERD. The lean chicken provides protein, while the whole grain noodles and mushrooms add fiber and essential nutrients.

10. Vegetable And Lentil Stew With Lean Lamb And Quinoa

Ingredients:
- 1 pound lean lamb shoulder or leg, cut into small pieces
- 1 cup dried green or brown lentils, rinsed and drained
- 2 cups mixed vegetables (such as carrots, potatoes, zucchini, and spinach)
- 2 cups low-sodium vegetable broth
- 1 cup quinoa
- 1 large onion, chopped
- 2 cloves garlic, minced
- 1 teaspoon dried rosemary
- Salt and pepper, to taste

Instructions:
1. In a large pot, sauté the lamb, onion, and garlic in a little water until the lamb is browned.
2. Add the lentils, mixed vegetables, vegetable broth, quinoa, and rosemary.
3. Bring to a boil, then reduce heat and simmer for 25-30 minutes or until the lentils and quinoa are tender.
4. Season with salt and pepper to taste.
5. Serve hot, garnished with fresh herbs (optional).

Tip:
- Use lean lamb to reduce fat content.

- Choose low-sodium vegetable broth to reduce acidity.
- Select quinoa as a whole grain to increase fiber content.
- Avoid adding spicy or acidic ingredients, which can trigger GERD symptoms.
- Cook slowly and gently to prevent acid reflux.

This recipe is gentle on the stomach and esophagus, making it suitable for those with GERD. The lean lamb provides protein, while the lentils, quinoa, and vegetables add fiber and essential nutrients.

Desserts

1. Fresh Fruit Salad With Low-Fat Yogurt

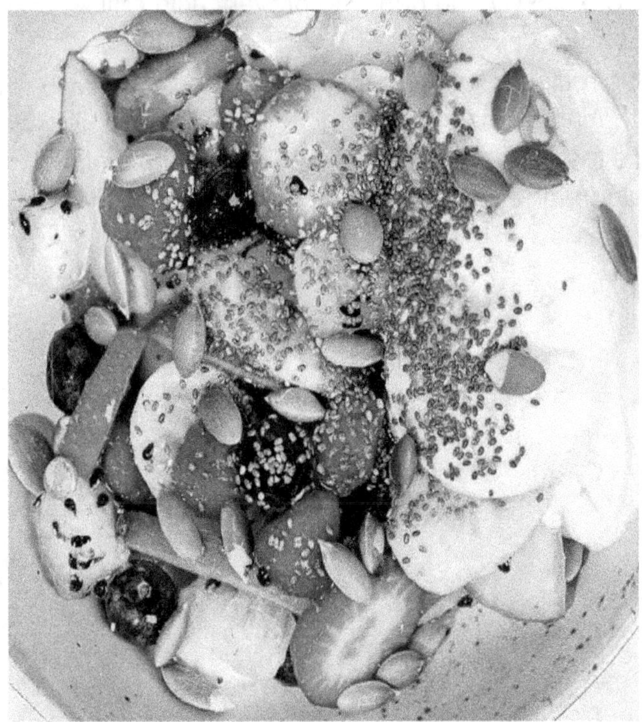

Fresh fruit salad with low-fat yogurt is a great option for a GERD-friendly snack or dessert. The fresh fruit provides natural sweetness and fiber, while the low-fat yogurt adds protein and creaminess without excessive fat.

Ingredients:

- 1 cup mixed fresh fruit (such as strawberries, blueberries, grapes, banana, and pineapple)
- 1/2 cup low-fat yogurt (plain or flavored, depending on your preference)
- 1 tablespoon honey (optional)

Instructions:
1. In a bowl, mix together the fresh fruit.
2. In a separate bowl, whisk together the low-fat yogurt and honey (if using).
3. Pour the yogurt mixture over the fresh fruit and toss gently to combine.
4. Serve immediately and enjoy!

This fruit salad with low-fat yogurt is not only delicious, but it's also gentle on the stomach and esophagus, making it a great option for those with GERD. The fresh fruit provides natural acidity, while the low-fat yogurt helps to neutralize any potential acid reflux.

2. Almond Flavor Cookies With Low Sugar Jam

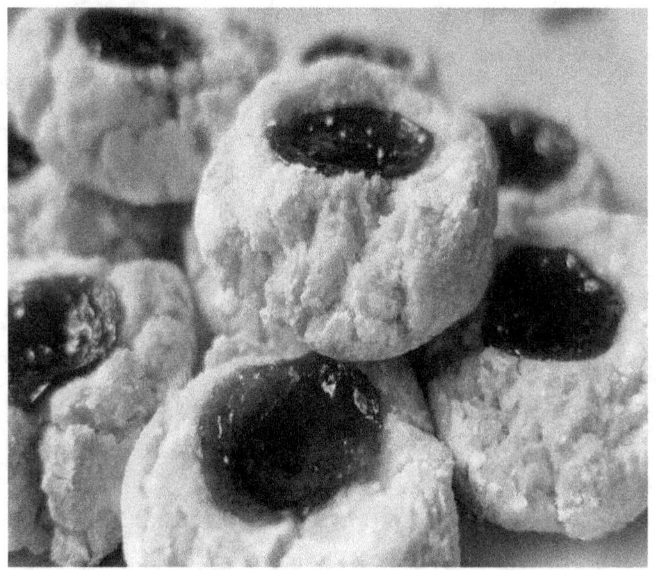

Almond flavor cookies with low sugar jam are a great option for a GERD-friendly snack. The almond flavor provides a delicious and subtle nutty taste, while the low sugar jam reduces the acidity and sugar content.

Ingredients:
- 1 1/2 cups all-purpose flour
- 1/2 cup almond flour
- 1/4 cup low sugar jam
- 1/4 cup unsalted butter, softened
- 1 egg
- 1 teaspoon almond extract
- Pinch of salt

Instructions:

1. Preheat the oven to 375°F (190°C). Line a baking sheet with parchment paper.
2. In a medium bowl, whisk together flour, almond flour, and salt.
3. In a large bowl, cream together butter and low sugar jam. Add egg and almond extract; mix well.
4. Gradually add dry ingredients to wet ingredients; mix until a dough forms.
5. Scoop tablespoon-sized balls onto the prepared baking sheet, leaving space between each cookie.
6. Bake for 12-15 minutes or until lightly golden.
7. Let cool on the baking sheet for 5 minutes before transferring to a wire rack to cool completely.

The almond flavor provides a soothing and calming effect, while the low sugar jam reduces the acidity and sugar content.

3. Ginger Panna Cotta With Low-Fat Cream

Ginger panna cotta with low-fat cream is a great option for a GERD-friendly treat. The ginger provides natural anti-inflammatory properties, while the low-fat cream reduces the acidity and fat content.

Ingredients:

- 1 cup low-fat cream
- 1/2 cup whole milk
- 1/4 cup granulated sugar

- 1-inch piece of fresh ginger, peeled and grated
- 1 teaspoon vanilla extract

Instructions:
1. In a medium saucepan, combine cream, milk, sugar, and grated ginger. Heat over medium heat, stirring occasionally, until sugar dissolves and mixture simmers.
2. Remove from heat and let steep for 10-15 minutes, allowing the ginger flavor to infuse.
3. Strain the mixture through a fine-mesh sieve into a clean bowl, discarding the ginger.
4. Whisk in vanilla extract.
5. Pour into individual serving cups or a large serving dish.
6. Refrigerate until set, about 4 hours or overnight.

The ginger provides natural anti-inflammatory properties, while the low-fat cream reduces the acidity and fat content.

4. Berry Sorbet With Low Sugar Content

Berry sorbet with low sugar content is a great option for a GERD-friendly dessert. The berries provide natural sweetness and antioxidants, while the low sugar content reduces the acidity and sugar load.
Ingredients:

- 2 cups mixed berries (such as blueberries, strawberries, raspberries)
- 1/4 cup granulated sugar
- 1/4 cup water
- 1 tablespoon honey (optional)

Instructions:
1. In a blender or food processor, puree the berries until smooth.
2. In a medium saucepan, combine the berry puree, sugar, and water. Heat over medium heat, stirring occasionally, until the sugar dissolves.
3. Remove from heat and let cool to room temperature.
4. Stir in honey (if using).
5. Pour the mixture into an ice cream maker and churn according to the manufacturer's instructions.
6. Once frozen, scoop into bowls and enjoy!

Note: If you don't have an ice cream maker, you can also freeze the mixture in a shallow metal pan and blend it in a food processor once frozen solid.

This berry sorbet with low sugar content is a refreshing and gentle dessert option for those with GERD. The berries provide natural sweetness and antioxidants, while the low sugar content reduces the acidity and sugar load.

5. Oatmeal Raisin Cookies With Low-Fat Milk

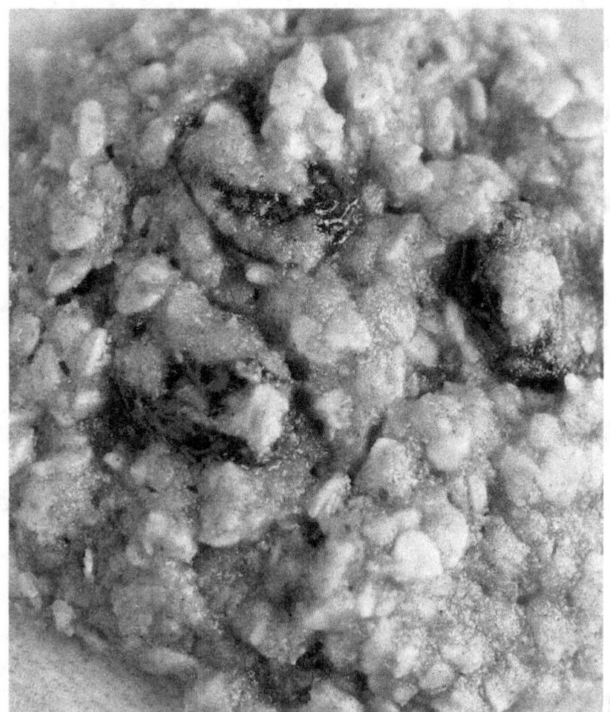

Oatmeal raisin cookies with low-fat milk are a great option for a GERD-friendly snack. The oatmeal provides fiber and a soothing effect, while the low-fat milk reduces the acidity and fat content.

Ingredients:
- 2 cups all-purpose flour
- 1 cup rolled oats
- 1/2 cup low-fat milk
- 1/4 cup sugar
- 1/4 cup brown sugar

- 1/2 cup raisins
- 1/2 teaspoon baking soda
- 1/2 teaspoon cinnamon
- 1/4 teaspoon nutmeg
- 1/4 teaspoon salt
- 1/4 cup unsalted butter, softened

Instructions:
1. Preheat the oven to 375°F (190°C). Line a baking sheet with parchment paper.
2. In a large bowl, whisk together flour, oats, sugar, brown sugar, baking soda, cinnamon, nutmeg, and salt.
3. In a separate bowl, whisk together low-fat milk and softened butter.
4. Add the wet ingredients to the dry ingredients and stir until a dough forms. Fold in raisins.
5. Scoop tablespoon-sized balls onto the prepared baking sheet, leaving space between each cookie.
6. Bake for 10-12 minutes or until lightly golden.
7. Let cool on the baking sheet for 5 minutes before transferring to a wire rack to cool completely.

The oatmeal provides fiber and a soothing effect, while the low-fat milk reduces the acidity and fat content.

6. Banana Pudding With Low-Fat Milk And Whole Grain Crackers

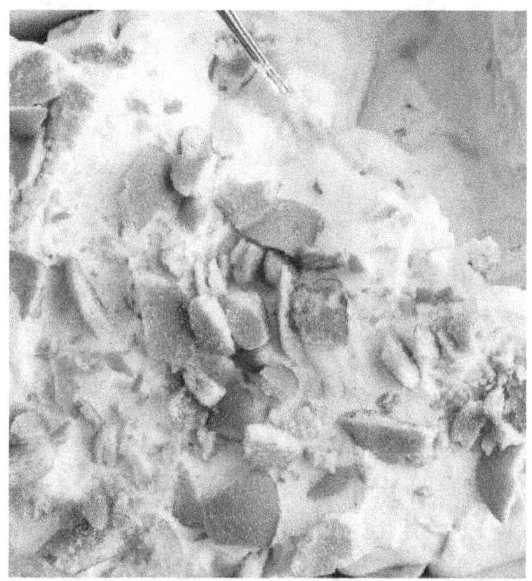

Banana pudding with low-fat milk and whole grain crackers is a great option for a GERD-friendly treat. The bananas provide natural sweetness and a soothing effect, while the low-fat milk reduces the acidity and fat content. The whole grain crackers add a satisfying crunch and fiber.

Ingredients:
- 4 ripe bananas
- 1 cup low-fat milk
- 2 tablespoons cornstarch
- 1/4 cup sugar
- 1/4 teaspoon salt
- 1/2 teaspoon vanilla extract
- 6-8 whole grain crackers

Instructions:

1. In a medium saucepan, whisk together milk, cornstarch, sugar, and salt. Cook over medium heat, stirring constantly, until the mixture thickens.
2. Remove from heat and stir in vanilla extract.
3. Slice the bananas into the pudding mixture and stir until well combined.
4. Pour into individual serving cups or a large serving dish.
5. Serve with whole grain crackers on the side.

The bananas provide natural sweetness and a soothing effect, while the low-fat milk reduces the acidity and fat content. The whole grain crackers add a satisfying crunch and fiber.

7. Lemon Bars With Whole Grain Crust And Low Sugar Filling

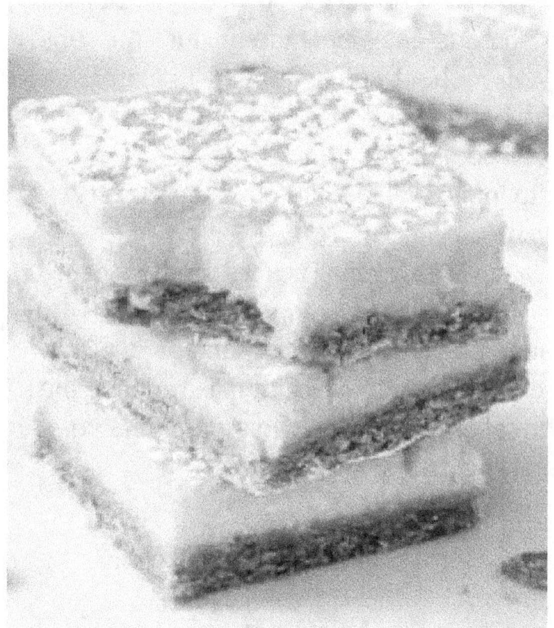

Lemon bars with whole grain crust and low sugar filling are a great option for a GERD-friendly dessert. The whole grain crust provides fiber and a satisfying crunch, while the low sugar filling reduces the acidity and sugar content.

Ingredients:
- 1 1/2 cups whole grain flour
- 1/2 cup granulated sugar
- 1/4 cup confectioners' sugar
- 1/2 cup unsalted butter, softened
- 2 large eggs
- 1 teaspoon grated lemon zest

- 2 tablespoons freshly squeezed lemon juice

Instructions:
1. Preheat the oven to 350°F (180°C). Line an 8-inch square baking dish with parchment paper.
2. In a medium bowl, whisk together flour, granulated sugar, and confectioners' sugar. Add softened butter and mix until a crumbly dough forms.
3. Press the dough into the prepared baking dish.
4. Bake for 20-22 minutes or until lightly golden.
5. While the crust is baking, whisk together eggs, lemon zest, and lemon juice.
6. When the crust is ready, pour the lemon mixture over the warm crust.
7. Bake for an additional 20-22 minutes or until the filling is set.
8. Let cool completely before slicing and serving.

These bars are gentle on the stomach and esophagus, making them a great option for those with GERD. The whole grain crust provides fiber and a satisfying crunch, while the low sugar filling reduces the acidity and sugar content.

8. Rice Pudding With Low-Fat Milk And Cinnamon

Rice pudding with low-fat milk and cinnamon is a great option for a GERD-friendly treat. The rice provides a gentle, easy-to-digest carbohydrate source, while the low-fat milk reduces the acidity and fat content. The cinnamon adds a warm, comforting flavor without triggering any acidic or spicy triggers.

Ingredients:
- 1 cup uncooked white rice
- 3 cups low-fat milk
- 1/4 cup granulated sugar
- 1/2 teaspoon ground cinnamon
- 1/4 teaspoon salt

Instructions:
1. In a medium saucepan, combine rice, milk, sugar, cinnamon, and salt.
2. Cook over medium heat, stirring constantly, until the rice is tender and the mixture thickens.
3. Remove from heat and let cool to room temperature.
4. Serve warm or chilled, depending on your preference.

The rice provides a gentle, easy-to-digest carbohydrate source, while the low-fat milk reduces the acidity and fat content. The cinnamon adds a warm, comforting flavor without triggering any acidic or spicy triggers.

9. Apple Crisp With Whole Grain Oats And Low Sugar Content

Apple Crisp with whole grain oats and low sugar content is a great option for a GERD-friendly treat. The apples provide a natural sweetness and fiber, while the whole grain oats add a satisfying crunch and more fiber. The low sugar content reduces the acidity and sugar load.

Ingredients:
- 6-8 medium apples, peeled and sliced
- 1/2 cup whole grain oats
- 1/4 cup brown sugar
- 1/4 cup granulated sugar
- 1/2 teaspoon cinnamon
- 1/4 teaspoon nutmeg
- 1/4 teaspoon salt
- 1/4 cup unsalted butter, melted

Instructions:
1. Preheat the oven to 375°F (190°C).
2. In a large mixing bowl, combine sliced apples, cinnamon, nutmeg, and salt.
3. In a separate bowl, mix together whole grain oats, brown sugar, and granulated sugar.
4. Add the melted butter to the oat mixture and stir until crumbly.
5. Pour the apple mixture into a 9x9-inch baking dish and top with the oat mixture.
6. Bake for 30-35 minutes or until the apples are tender and the topping is golden brown.

7. Serve warm, topped with a dollop of low-fat whipped cream or vanilla ice cream (optional).

The apples provide a natural sweetness and fiber, while the whole grain oats add a satisfying crunch and more fiber. The low sugar content reduces the acidity and sugar load.

10. Chia Seeds Pudding With Low-Fat Coconut Milk And Fresh Fruit

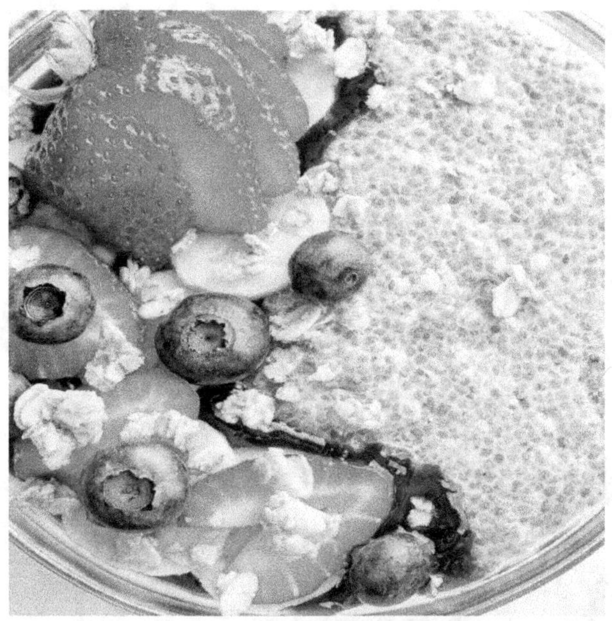

Chia Seeds pudding with low-fat coconut milk and fresh fruit is a great option for a GERD-friendly treat. The chia seeds provide a boost of omega-3

fatty acids and fiber, while the low-fat coconut milk reduces the acidity and fat content. The fresh fruit adds natural sweetness and flavor.

Ingredients:
- 1/2 cup chia seeds
- 1 cup low-fat coconut milk
- 1 tablespoon honey or maple syrup (optional)
- 1/2 cup fresh fruit (such as berries, sliced mango, or diced pineapple)

Instructions:
1. In a small bowl, mix together chia seeds and low-fat coconut milk. Let it sit for 5-10 minutes until the chia seeds absorb the liquid and form a gel-like texture.
2. Add honey or maple syrup if desired for sweetness.
3. Top with fresh fruit and serve chilled.

The chia seeds provide a boost of omega-3 fatty acids and fiber, while the low-fat coconut milk reduces the acidity and fat content. The fresh fruit adds natural sweetness and flavor without triggering any acidic or spicy triggers.

Appetizers

1. Grilled Chicken Skewers With Low-Fat Cocktail Sauce

Grilled chicken skewers with low-fat cocktail sauce are a great choice for a GERD-friendly meal. The grilled chicken provides lean protein, while the low-fat cocktail sauce reduces the acidity and fat content.

Ingredients:

- 1 pound boneless, skinless chicken breast or thighs, cut into 1-inch pieces
- 1/2 cup low-fat cocktail sauce
- 1/4 cup plain Greek yogurt
- 1 tablespoon lemon juice
- 1/2 teaspoon Dijon mustard
- 1/4 teaspoon paprika
- Salt and pepper, to taste
- 10-12 bamboo skewers, soaked in water for 30 minutes

Instructions:

1. Preheat the grill to medium-high heat.
2. Thread chicken pieces onto skewers.
3. Grill for 8-10 minutes, turning occasionally, until cooked through.
4. In a small bowl, mix together low-fat cocktail sauce, Greek yogurt, lemon juice, Dijon mustard, paprika, salt, and pepper.

5. Serve grilled chicken skewers with low-fat cocktail sauce for dipping.

2. Vegetable Spring Rolls With Whole Grain Wrappers

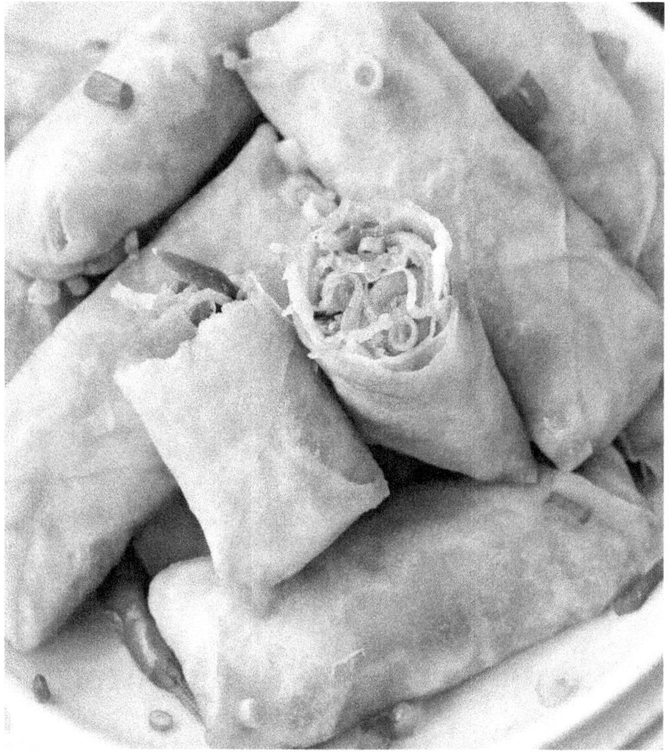

Vegetable spring rolls with whole grain wrappers are a great option for a GERD-friendly meal. The whole grain wrappers provide fiber and a satisfying crunch, while the vegetables add natural sweetness and flavor without triggering any acidic or spicy triggers.

Ingredients:

- 1 package whole grain spring roll wrappers
- 1/2 cup shredded carrots
- 1/2 cup shredded cabbage
- 1/2 cup shredded cucumber
- 1/4 cup chopped scallions
- 1/4 cup chopped fresh mint leaves
- 2 tablespoons low-sodium soy sauce (optional)

Instructions:

1. Fill a large bowl with warm water.
2. Place a whole grain wrapper in the water for 10-15 seconds until soft and pliable.
3. Place the wrapper on a clean surface and add shredded vegetables and herbs in the center.
4. Fold the bottom half over the filling, then fold in sides and roll up tightly.
5. Repeat with remaining wrappers and filling ingredients.
6. Serve with low-sodium soy sauce for dipping (if desired).

3. Lentil And Vegetable Fritters With Low-Fat Tzatziki Sauce

A flavorful and healthy option. Lentil and Vegetable fritters with low-fat Tzatziki sauce are a great choice for a GERD-friendly meal. The lentils and vegetables provide fiber and protein, while the low-fat Tzatziki sauce reduces the acidity and fat content.

Ingredients:
- 1 cup cooked lentils
- 1 cup mixed vegetables (such as carrots, zucchini, and onions)
- 1/2 cup whole grain breadcrumbs
- 1 egg
- 1/4 cup low-fat plain Greek yogurt
- 1/4 cup diced cucumber
- 1 tablespoon lemon juice
- 1/2 teaspoon garlic powder
- Salt and pepper to taste

Instructions:
1. In a bowl, mix together lentils, vegetables, breadcrumbs, egg, and spices.
2. Form into patties and cook in a non-stick skillet until golden brown.
3. In a separate bowl, mix together Greek yogurt, cucumber, lemon juice, garlic powder, salt, and pepper.
4. Serve fritters with low-fat Tzatziki sauce for dipping.

4. Grilled Chicken Satay With Whole Grain Bread And Peanut Sauce

A flavorful and nutritious option. Grilled chicken satay with whole grain bread and peanut sauce is a great choice for a GERD-friendly meal. The grilled chicken provides lean protein, whole grain bread offers fiber and a satisfying crunch, and the peanut sauce adds creaminess without excessive acidity or spice.

Ingredients:
- 1 pound boneless, skinless chicken breast or thighs, cut into skewers
- 1/2 cup whole grain bread, cut into slices
- 1/2 cup peanut sauce (made with low-fat peanut butter, Greek yogurt, and honey)
- 1/4 cup low-fat coconut milk
- 2 tablespoons soy sauce (low-sodium)
- 2 tablespoons honey
- 1 tablespoon grated ginger
- 1/4 teaspoon red pepper flakes (optional)

Instructions:
1. Grill chicken skewers until cooked through.
2. Toast whole grain bread slices.
3. In a bowl, mix together peanut sauce ingredients.
4. Serve grilled chicken satay with whole grain bread and peanut sauce for dipping.

5. Steamed Mussels With Whole Grain Bread And Low-Fat Garlic Butter

Steamed mussels with whole grain bread and low-fat garlic butter are great choices for a GERD-friendly meal. The mussels provide lean protein, whole grain bread offers fiber and a satisfying crunch, and the low-fat garlic butter adds flavor without excessive acidity or fat.

Ingredients:
- 2 pounds mussels, scrubbed and debearded
- 2 slices whole grain bread
- 2 tablespoons low-fat butter
- 1 clove garlic, minced
- 1/4 cup white wine (optional)
- 1/4 cup low-sodium chicken broth
- Salt and pepper to taste

Instructions:
1. Steam mussels until opened.
2. Toast whole grain bread slices.
3. Mix low-fat butter, garlic, and a pinch of salt and pepper.
4. Serve steamed mussels with whole grain bread and low-fat garlic butter for dipping.

6. Roasted Vegetables Tarts With Whole Grain Crust And Low-Fat Cheese

Roasted Vegetable tarts with whole grain crust and low-fat cheese are great choices for a GERD-friendly meal. The whole grain crust provides fiber and a satisfying crunch, the roasted vegetables add natural sweetness and flavor, and the low-fat cheese reduces the acidity and fat content.

Ingredients:
- 1 cup whole grain flour
- 1/2 cup low-fat butter, chilled and cubed
- 1/2 cup ice-cold water
- 2 cups mixed roasted vegetables (such as sweet potatoes, Brussels sprouts, and caramelized onions)
- 1/2 cup low-fat cheese, shredded (such as mozzarella or feta)
- Salt and pepper to taste

Instructions:
1. Preheat the oven to 375°F (190°C).
2. Make the whole grain crust by mixing flour, butter, and ice-cold water.
3. Roll out the dough and place in a tart pan.
4. Fill with roasted vegetables and top with low-fat cheese.
5. Bake for 25-30 minutes or until the crust is golden brown and the cheese is melted.

This meal is gentle on the stomach and esophagus, making it a great option for those with GERD. The whole grain crust provides fiber and a satisfying crunch, the roasted vegetables add natural sweetness and flavor, and the low-fat cheese reduces the acidity and fat content.

7. Spinach And Artichoke Dip With Whole Grain Pita Chips

Spinach and artichoke dip with whole grain pita chips are a great choice for a GERD-friendly snack. The spinach and artichoke dip provides a creamy and flavorful base without excessive acidity or spice, while the whole grain pita chips offer a satisfying crunch and fiber.

Ingredients:
- 1 cup cooked spinach
- 1 cup artichoke hearts
- 1 cup low-fat cream cheese
- 1/2 cup low-fat mayonnaise
- 1/4 cup chopped fresh parsley
- 1/2 teaspoon lemon juice
- Salt and pepper to taste
- 1 bag whole grain pita chips

Instructions:
1. Mix all ingredients except pita chips in a bowl until well combined.
2. Serve dip with whole grain pita chips.

The spinach and artichoke dip provides a creamy and flavorful base without excessive acidity or spice, while the whole grain pita chips offer a satisfying crunch and fiber.

8. Grilled Chicken Skewers With Low-Fat Balsamic Glaze

Grilled chicken skewers with low-fat balsamic glaze are a great choice for a GERD-friendly meal. The grilled chicken provides lean protein, while the low-fat balsamic glaze adds a sweet and tangy flavor without excessive acidity or fat.

Ingredients:
- 1 pound boneless, skinless chicken breast or thighs, cut into skewers
- 1/4 cup low-fat balsamic glaze (made with reduced balsamic vinegar and honey)
- 2 tablespoons olive oil
- 2 cloves garlic, minced
- 1 teaspoon dried thyme
- Salt and pepper to taste

Instructions:
1. Preheat the grill to medium-high heat.
2. In a bowl, whisk together balsamic glaze, olive oil, garlic, thyme, salt, and pepper.
3. Add chicken skewers and marinate for at least 30 minutes.
4. Grill chicken skewers until cooked through, brushing with additional balsamic glaze during cooking.

9. Chicken And Vegetable Meatballs With Whole Grain Bread And Low-Fat Marinara Sauce

Chicken and Vegetable meatballs with whole grain bread and low-fat Marinara sauce are great choices for a GERD-friendly meal. The meatballs provide lean protein and fiber, while the whole grain bread offers additional fiber and a satisfying crunch. The low-fat Marinara sauce adds flavor without excessive acidity or fat.

Ingredients:

- 1 pound ground chicken
- 1/2 cup finely chopped vegetables (such as onions, carrots, and bell peppers)
- 1 egg
- 1/2 cup whole grain breadcrumbs
- 1 cup low-fat Marinara sauce
- 4 slices whole grain bread

Instructions:

1. Preheat the oven to 400°F (200°C).
2. Mix meatball ingredients in a bowl until well combined.
3. Form into balls and bake for 15-20 minutes or until cooked through.
4. Serve with whole grain bread and low-fat Marinara sauce for dipping.

10. Steamed Dumplings With Whole Grain Wrappers And Low-Fat Dipping Sauce

Steamed dumplings with whole grain wrappers and low-fat dipping sauce are a great choice for a GERD-friendly meal. The whole grain wrappers provide fiber and a satisfying texture, while the steamed dumplings offer a gentle and easily digestible protein source. The low-fat dipping sauce adds flavor without excessive acidity or fat.

Ingredients:
- 1 package whole grain dumpling wrappers
- 1/2 cup ground chicken or turkey
- 1/2 cup finely chopped vegetables (such as cabbage and carrots)
- 2 tablespoons low-fat soy sauce
- 2 tablespoons low-fat vinegar
- 1 tablespoon honey
- 1/4 cup water

Instructions:
1. Mix dumpling filling ingredients in a bowl until well combined.
2. Place a small spoonful of filling in the center of each wrapper.
3. Steam dumplings until cooked through.
4. Mix dipping sauce ingredients in a bowl until well combined.
5. Serve steamed dumplings with low-fat dipping sauce.

Snacks

1. Fresh Fruit With Almond Butter On Whole Grain Crackers

Fresh fruit with almond butter on whole grain crackers is a great choice for a GERD-friendly snack. The fresh fruit provides natural sweetness and fiber, while the almond butter adds healthy fats and protein. The whole grain crackers offer additional fiber and a satisfying crunch.

Ingredients:
- 1 cup fresh fruit (such as apples, bananas, or berries)
- 2 tablespoons almond butter
- 4-6 whole grain crackers

Instructions:
1. Spread almond butter on whole grain crackers.
2. Top with fresh fruit.
3. Serve and enjoy!

This snack is gentle on the stomach and esophagus, making it a great option for those with GERD. The fresh fruit provides natural sweetness and fiber, while the almond butter adds healthy fats and protein. The whole grain crackers offer additional fiber and a satisfying crunch.

2. Low-Fat Yogurt With Honey And Whole Grain Granola

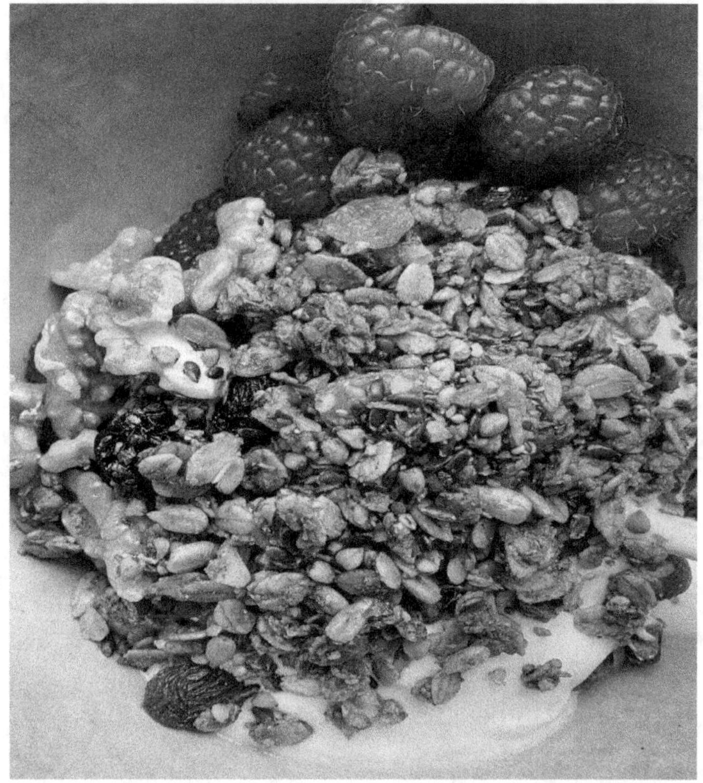

Low-fat yogurt with honey and whole grain granola is a great choice for a GERD-friendly snack. The low-fat yogurt provides protein and calcium, while the honey adds natural sweetness without excessive acidity. The whole grain granola offers fiber and a satisfying crunch.

Ingredients:

- 1 cup low-fat yogurt

- 1 tablespoon honey
- 2 tablespoons whole grain granola

Instructions:
1. Mix yogurt and honey in a bowl until well combined.
2. Top with whole grain granola.
3. Serve and enjoy!

The low-fat yogurt provides protein and calcium, while the honey adds natural sweetness without excessive acidity. The whole grain granola offers fiber and a satisfying crunch.

3. Veggie Sticks With Low-Fat Ranch Dip

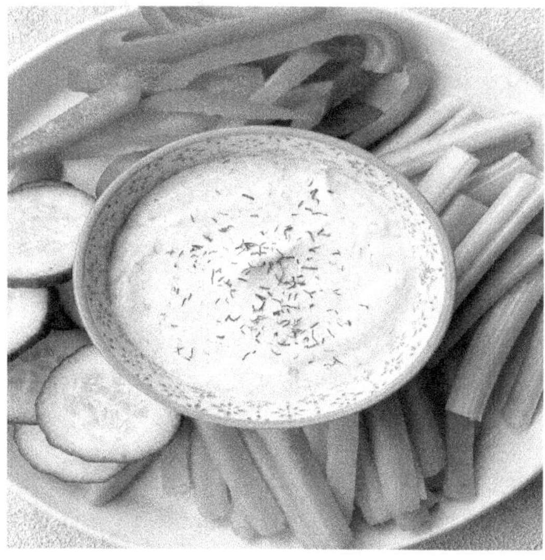

A crunchy and delicious snack. Veggie sticks with low-fat ranch dip are a great choice for a GERD-friendly snack. The veggie sticks provide fiber and vitamins, while the low-fat ranch dip adds a creamy and tangy flavor without excessive acidity or fat.

Ingredients:
- 1 cup mixed veggie sticks (such as carrots, cucumbers, and bell peppers)
- 1/2 cup low-fat ranch dip (made with low-fat sour cream and herbs)

Instructions:
1. Serve veggie sticks with low-fat ranch dip for a healthy and tasty snack.

The veggie sticks provide fiber and vitamins, while the low-fat ranch dip adds a creamy and tangy flavor without excessive acidity or fat.

4. Whole Grain Toast With Avocado And Tomato

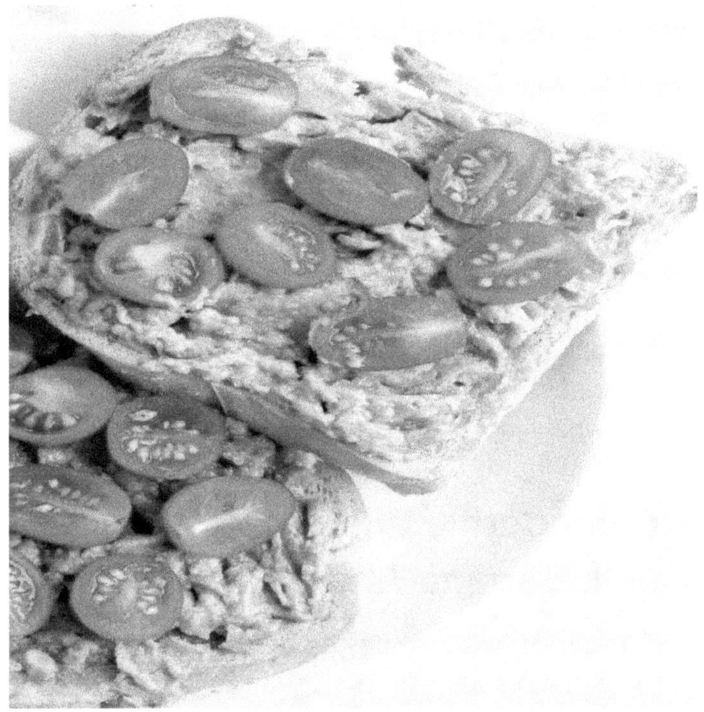

A nutritious and delicious snack. Whole grain toast with avocado and tomato is a great choice for a GERD-friendly snack. The whole grain toast provides fiber and a satisfying crunch, while the avocado adds healthy fats and creaminess. The tomato adds natural sweetness and acidity without being too overwhelming.

Ingredients:

- 2 slices whole grain bread
- 1 ripe avocado, mashed

- 1 tomato, sliced
- Salt and pepper to taste

Instructions:
1. Toast whole grain bread until lightly browned.
2. Spread mashed avocado on top.
3. Add sliced tomato.
4. Season with salt and pepper to taste.
5. Serve and enjoy!

The whole grain toast provides fiber and a satisfying crunch, while the avocado adds healthy fats and creaminess. The tomato adds natural sweetness and acidity without being too overwhelming.

5. Smoothie With Low-Fat Milk,Banana And Spinach

The low-fat milk provides protein and calcium, while the banana adds natural sweetness and creamy texture. The spinach adds a boost of antioxidants and fiber without overwhelming the palate.
Ingredients:
- 1 cup low-fat milk
- 1 ripe banana
- 1 cup fresh spinach leaves
- 1 tablespoon honey (optional)

Instructions:
1. Blend all ingredients in a blender until smooth.

2. Add honey to taste, if desired.
3. Serve and enjoy.

6. Roasted Chickpeas With Whole Grain Seasoning

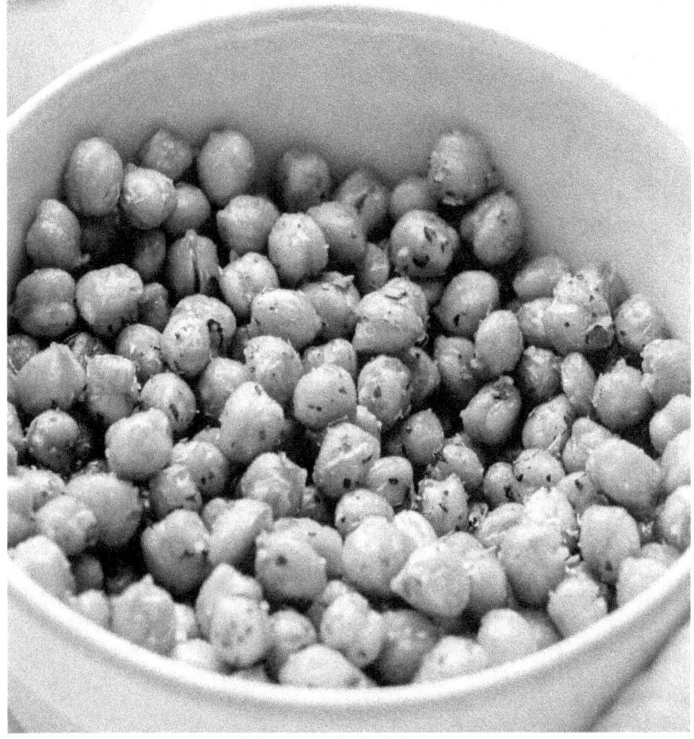

Roasted chickpeas with whole grain seasoning are a great choice for a GERD-friendly snack. The chickpeas provide protein and fiber, while the whole grain seasoning adds a boost of fiber and nutrients without excessive acidity or spice.
Ingredients:

- 1 can chickpeas
- 2 tablespoons whole grain seasoning (such as paprika, garlic powder, and onion powder)
- 1 tablespoon olive oil
- Salt and pepper to taste

Instructions:
1. Preheat the oven to 400°F (200°C).
2. Rinse chickpeas and remove any excess water.
3. Mix chickpeas with olive oil, whole grain seasoning, salt, and pepper.
4. Spread on a baking sheet and roast for 30-40 minutes or until crispy.
5. Serve and enjoy.

7. Cottage Cheese With Fresh Fruit And Whole Grain Crackers

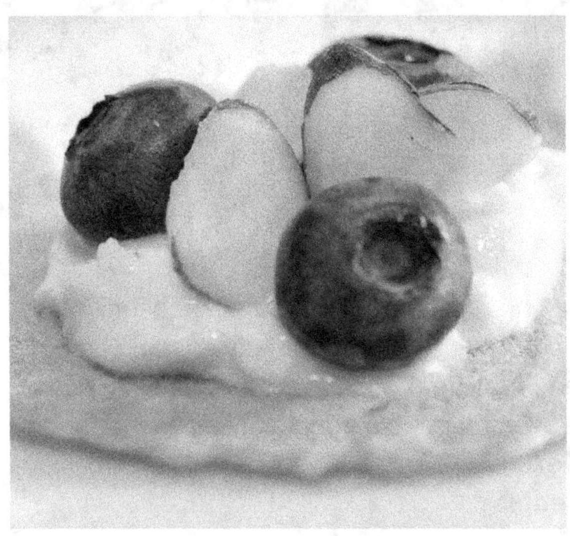

Cottage cheese with fresh fruit and whole grain crackers is a great choice for a GERD-friendly snack. The cottage cheese provides protein and calcium, while the fresh fruit adds natural sweetness and fiber. The whole grain crackers offer additional fiber and a satisfying crunch.

Ingredients:
- 1 cup cottage cheese
- 1/2 cup fresh fruit (such as berries, sliced peaches, or diced pineapple)
- 4-6 whole grain crackers

Instructions:
1. Mix cottage cheese and fresh fruit in a bowl.
2. Serve with whole grain crackers on the side.
3. Enjoy as a healthy and satisfying snack!

8. Hard-Boiled Eggs With Whole Grain Toast

A classic and satisfying snack. Hard-boiled eggs with whole grain toast are a great choice for a GERD-friendly snack. The hard-boiled eggs provide protein and a comforting bite, while the whole grain toast offers fiber and a satisfying crunch.

Ingredients:
- 2 eggs
- 2 slices whole grain bread
- Salt and pepper to taste

Instructions:

1. Boil eggs for 10-12 minutes or until cooked through.
2. Toast whole grain bread until lightly browned.
3. Serve eggs with whole grain toast and a sprinkle of salt and pepper.
4. Enjoy as a comforting and protein-rich snack.

9. Apple Slices With Almond Butter And Whole Grain Crackers

Apple slices with almond butter and whole grain crackers are great choices for a GERD-friendly snack. The apple slices provide a natural sweetness and fiber, while the almond butter adds healthy fats and protein. The whole grain crackers offer additional fiber and a satisfying crunch.

Ingredients:
- 1 apple, sliced
- 2 tablespoons almond butter
- 4-6 whole grain crackers

Instructions:
1. Spread almond butter on apple slices.
2. Serve with whole grain crackers on the side.
3. Enjoy as a healthy and satisfying snack!

10. Carrot Sticks With Hummus And Whole Grain Pita Chips

Carrot sticks with hummus and whole grain pita chips are great choices for a GERD-friendly snack. The carrot sticks provide a crunchy and sweet snack, while the hummus adds a creamy and protein-rich dip. The whole grain pita chips offer additional fiber and a satisfying crunch.

Ingredients:
- 4-6 carrot sticks
- 1/2 cup hummus
- 4-6 whole grain pita chips

Instructions:
1. Serve carrot sticks with hummus for dipping.
2. Enjoy with whole grain pita chips on the side.
3. Snack on and enjoy.

Smoothies

1. Banana-Avocado Smoothie

The Banana-Avocado Smoothie is a great choice for a GERD-friendly drink. The banana provides natural sweetness and a soothing effect on the stomach, while the avocado adds healthy fats and creaminess. The combination of the two ingredients creates a smooth and velvety texture that is gentle on the esophagus.

Ingredients:
- 1 ripe banana
- 1 ripe avocado
- 1/2 cup almond milk or low-fat milk
- 1 tablespoon honey (optional)
- Ice cubes (optional)

Instructions:
1. Peel the banana and avocado and add them to a blender.
2. Add the almond milk and honey (if using) to the blender.
3. Blend the mixture until smooth and creamy.
4. Add ice cubes (if using) and blend until the ice is crushed and the smoothie is the desired consistency.
5. Pour into a glass and serve immediately.

2. Berry Bliss Smoothie

The Berry Bliss Smoothie is a great choice for a GERD-friendly drink. The mixed berries provide a natural sweetness and a boost of antioxidants, while the low-fat yogurt adds protein and a soothing effect on the stomach. The spinach adds a boost of fiber and antioxidants without overpowering the flavor of the berries.

Ingredients:
- 1 cup mixed berries (such as blueberries, strawberries, raspberries)
- 1/2 cup low-fat yogurt
- 1 handful of fresh spinach leaves

- 1/2 cup almond milk or low-fat milk
- 1 tablespoon honey (optional)
- Ice cubes (optional)

Instructions:
1. Add the mixed berries, low-fat yogurt, spinach, and almond milk to a blender.
2. Blend the mixture until smooth and creamy.
3. Add honey (if using) and blend until well combined.
4. Add ice cubes (if using) and blend until the ice is crushed and the smoothie is the desired consistency.
5. Pour into a glass and serve immediately.

3. Citrus Refresher Smoothie

The Citrus Refresher Smoothie is a great choice for a GERD-friendly drink. The combination of citrus fruits provides a natural sweetness and a boost of vitamin C, while the low-fat yogurt adds protein and a soothing effect on the stomach.
Ingredients:
- 1/2 cup freshly squeezed orange juice
- 1/2 cup freshly squeezed grapefruit juice
- 1/4 cup freshly squeezed pineapple juice
- 1/2 cup low-fat yogurt
- 1 tablespoon honey (optional)
- Ice cubes (optional)

Instructions:

1. Add the citrus juices and low-fat yogurt to a blender.
2. Blend the mixture until smooth and creamy.
3. Add honey (if using) and blend until well combined.
4. Add ice cubes (if using) and blend until the ice is crushed and the smoothie is the desired consistency.
5. Pour into a glass and serve immediately.

Note: Be sure to use freshly squeezed juices and not concentrated or bottled juices, which can be high in acidity and trigger GERD symptoms. Also, start with a small amount and adjust to taste, as citrus fruits can be triggering for some individuals with GERD.

4. Ginger Zinger Smoothie

The Ginger Zinger Smoothie is a great choice for a GERD-friendly drink. The ginger provides a natural anti-inflammatory effect and can help reduce nausea and inflammation in the esophagus, while the pineapple and coconut water add a refreshing and soothing effect.

Ingredients:
- 1-inch piece of fresh ginger, peeled and grated
- 1 cup pineapple chunks
- 1 cup coconut water
- 1/2 cup low-fat yogurt
- 1 tablespoon honey (optional)
- Ice cubes (optional)

Instructions:
1. Add the ginger, pineapple, coconut water, and low-fat yogurt to a blender.
2. Blend the mixture until smooth and creamy.
3. Add honey (if using) and blend until well combined.
4. Add ice cubes (if using) and blend until the ice is crushed and the smoothie is the desired consistency.
5. Pour into a glass and serve immediately.

This smoothie is a great option, as it is easy to digest and can help reduce inflammation in the esophagus. The ginger provides a natural anti-inflammatory effect, while the pineapple and coconut water add a refreshing and soothing effect.

Note: Start with a small amount of ginger (1/2 inch) and adjust to taste, as ginger can be overpowering for some individuals. Also, be sure to use fresh ginger and not ginger powder or supplements, which can be more potent and triggering for GERD symptoms.

5. Mango Peach Delight Smoothie

The Mango Peach Delight Smoothie is a great choice for a GERD-friendly drink. The mango and peach provide a natural sweetness and a soothing effect on the stomach, while the low-fat yogurt adds protein and a creamy texture.

Ingredients:
- 1 ripe mango, diced
- 1 ripe peach, diced
- 1/2 cup low-fat yogurt
- 1/2 cup almond milk or low-fat milk
- 1 tablespoon honey (optional)
- Ice cubes (optional)

Instructions:
1. Add the mango, peach, low-fat yogurt, and almond milk to a blender.
2. Blend the mixture until smooth and creamy.
3. Add honey (if using) and blend until well combined.
4. Add ice cubes (if using) and blend until the ice is crushed and the smoothie is the desired consistency.
5. Pour into a glass and serve immediately.

Note: Be sure to use ripe mango and peach, as unripe fruit can be high in acidity and trigger GERD symptoms. Also, start with a small amount and adjust to taste, as some individuals with GERD may need to limit their fruit intake.

6. Pina Colada Smoothie

A creamy and tropical smoothie. The Pina Colada Smoothie is a great choice for a GERD-friendly drink. The pineapple and coconut milk provide a natural sweetness and a soothing effect on the stomach, while the low-fat yogurt adds protein and a creamy texture.

Ingredients:
- 1 cup pineapple chunks
- 1/2 cup coconut milk
- 1/2 cup low-fat yogurt
- 1 tablespoon honey (optional)
- Ice cubes (optional)

Instructions:
1. Add the pineapple, coconut milk, and low-fat yogurt to a blender.
2. Blend the mixture until smooth and creamy.
3. Add honey (if using) and blend until well combined.
4. Add ice cubes (if using) and blend until the ice is crushed and the smoothie is the desired consistency.
5. Pour into a glass and serve immediately.

Note: Be sure to use low-fat coconut milk and yogurt to avoid triggering GERD symptoms. Also, start with a small amount and adjust to taste, as some individuals with GERD may need to limit their coconut intake.

7. Spinach Surprise Smoothie

The Spinach Surprise Smoothie is a great choice for a GERD-friendly drink. The spinach provides a boost of antioxidants and fiber, while the banana and almond milk add natural sweetness and a creamy texture.

Ingredients:
- 2 cups fresh spinach leaves
- 1 ripe banana
- 1 cup almond milk
- 1/2 cup low-fat yogurt
- 1 tablespoon honey (optional)
- Ice cubes (optional)

Instructions:
1. Add the spinach, banana, almond milk, and low-fat yogurt to a blender.
2. Blend the mixture until smooth and creamy.
3. Add honey (if using) and blend until well combined.
4. Add ice cubes (if using) and blend until the ice is crushed and the smoothie is the desired consistency.
5. Pour into a glass and serve immediately.

Note: Don't worry, the spinach won't overpower the flavor. The banana and almond milk will mask any bitter taste, leaving you with a delicious and healthy smoothie.

8. Strawberry Sunshine Smoothie

The Strawberry Sunshine Smoothie is a great choice for a GERD-friendly drink. The strawberries provide a natural sweetness and a boost of vitamin C, while the almond milk and low-fat yogurt add a creamy texture and a soothing effect on the stomach.

Ingredients:
- 1 cup fresh or frozen strawberries
- 1 cup almond milk
- 1/2 cup low-fat yogurt
- 1 tablespoon honey (optional)
- Ice cubes (optional)

Instructions:
1. Add the strawberries, almond milk, and low-fat yogurt to a blender.
2. Blend the mixture until smooth and creamy.
3. Add honey (if using) and blend until well combined.
4. Add ice cubes (if using) and blend until the ice is crushed and the smoothie is the desired consistency.
5. Pour into a glass and serve immediately.

Note: Be sure to use fresh or frozen strawberries, as strawberry juice or preserves can be high in acidity and trigger GERD symptoms. Also, start with a small amount and adjust to taste, as some individuals with GERD may need to limit their fruit intake.

9. Tropical Temptation Smoothie

The Tropical Temptation Smoothie is a great choice for a GERD-friendly drink. The combination of pineapple, mango, and coconut milk provides a natural sweetness and a creamy texture, while the spinach adds a boost of antioxidants and fiber.

Ingredients:
- 1 cup pineapple chunks
- 1 cup mango chunks
- 1/2 cup coconut milk
- 2 cups fresh spinach leaves
- 1/2 cup low-fat yogurt
- 1 tablespoon honey (optional)
- Ice cubes (optional)

Instructions:
1. Add the pineapple, mango, coconut milk, spinach, and low-fat yogurt to a blender.
2. Blend the mixture until smooth and creamy.
3. Add honey (if using) and blend until well combined.
4. Add ice cubes (if using) and blend until the ice is crushed and the smoothie is the desired consistency.
5. Pour into a glass and serve immediately.

Note: Be sure to use low-fat coconut milk and yogurt to avoid triggering GERD symptoms. Also, start with a small amount and adjust to taste, as some individuals with GERD may need to limit their coconut intake.

10. Vanilla Dream Smoothie

The Vanilla Dream Smoothie is a great choice for a GERD-friendly drink. The vanilla protein powder and almond milk provide a soothing and calming effect on the stomach, while the banana adds natural sweetness and a creamy texture.

Ingredients:
- 1 scoop vanilla protein powder
- 1 cup almond milk
- 1 ripe banana
- 1/2 cup low-fat yogurt
- 1 tablespoon honey (optional)
- Ice cubes (optional)

Instructions:
1. Add the protein powder, almond milk, banana, and low-fat yogurt to a blender.
2. Blend the mixture until smooth and creamy.
3. Add honey (if using) and blend until well combined.
4. Add ice cubes (if using) and blend until the ice is crushed and the smoothie is the desired consistency.
5. Pour into a glass and serve immediately.

Note: Be sure to use a low-fat protein powder and yogurt to avoid triggering GERD symptoms. Also, start with a small amount and adjust to taste, as some individuals with GERD may need to limit their protein intake.

Chapter Four

Lifestyle Changes

1. **Eat smaller,more frequent meals:** Reduce symptoms by not overloading the stomach with large meals.
2. **Avoid trigger foods:** Identify and avoid foods that trigger GERD symptoms.
3. **Raise the head of your bed:** Elevate the head of your bed by 6-8 inches to prevent acid reflux at night.
4. **Lose weight:** Excess weight can put pressure on the stomach, worsening GERD symptoms.
5. **Avoid tight clothing:** Wear loose, comfortable clothing to reduce pressure on the stomach.
6. **Manage stress:** Stress can exacerbate GERD symptoms; practice stress-reducing techniques like meditation or deep breathing.
7. **Quit smoking:** Smoking can worsen GERD symptoms; quitting can help alleviate them.
8. **Limit alcohol and caffeine:** Both can relax the lower esophageal sphincter, worsen GERD symptoms.
9. **Avoid lying down after eating:** Wait at least 2-3 hours after eating before lying down or going to bed.
10. **Consider keeping a food diary:** Tracking food intake and symptoms can help identify trigger foods and monitor progress.

Remember,everyone's triggers and symptoms are different, so it's essential to work with a healthcare provider to develop a personalized plan.

Healthy Eating Habits To Adopt

1. Eat slowly and mindfully
2. Avoid overeating
3. Choose smaller, more frequent meals
4. Select foods low in acidity and fat
5. Incorporate GERD-friendly foods like almonds, oatmeal, and ginger
6. Avoid lying down after eating
7. Wait 2-3 hours after eating before bedtime
8. Raise the head of your bed 6-8 inches
9. Keep a food diary to track triggers and symptoms
10. Stay hydrated with water and low-acidity beverages

Some specific foods to include in your diet are:
- Lean proteins like chicken, fish, and tofu
- Vegetables like green beans, carrots, and sweet potatoes
- Fruits like bananas, melons, and berries
- Whole grains like brown rice, quinoa, and whole-wheat bread
- Low-fat dairy products like milk, yogurt, and cheese

Stress Management Techniques

1. **Deep Breathing Exercises:** Slow, deliberate breathing can help calm the body and reduce stress.
2. **Progressive Muscle Relaxation:** Tensing and relaxing different muscle groups can release physical tension.
3. **Meditation and Mindfulness:** Focusing on the present moment can reduce stress and anxiety.
4. **Yoga:** Combining physical movement with deep breathing and meditation can help manage stress.
5. **Journaling:** Writing down thoughts and feelings can help process and release emotions.
6. **Visualization:** Imagining a peaceful, relaxing scene can help calm the mind and body.
7. **Walking and Exercise:** Regular physical activity can reduce stress and improve overall health.
8. **Grounding Techniques:** Focusing on the five senses can help bring the mind back to the present moment.
9. **Mindful Eating:** Eating slowly, savoring food, and avoiding screens during meals can help reduce stress and symptoms.
10. **Seek Support:** Talking to a therapist, support group, or loved ones can help manage stress and emotions.

Remember,everyone is unique and it's essential to experiment with different techniques to find what works best for you. Consult with a healthcare professional before starting any new stress management practices.

Exercises And Physical Activities

1. **Yoga:** Certain poses, like child's pose, downward-facing dog, and pigeon pose, can help strengthen the lower esophageal sphincter and improve digestion.
2. **Brisk Walking:** Regular walking can help reduce symptoms by improving digestion and reducing stress.
3. **Swimming:** This low-impact exercise can help strengthen the muscles without putting excessive strain on the stomach.
4. **Cycling:** Stationary cycling or using a recumbent bike can be a gentle way to improve cardiovascular health without exacerbating GERD.
5. **Stretching:** Gentle stretching exercises can help relieve tension and improve digestion.
6. **Low-Impact Aerobics:** Dancing, step aerobics, or low-impact cardio machines like ellipticals can be modified to suit individual comfort levels.
7. **Pelvic Floor Exercises:** Strengthening the pelvic floor muscles can help improve digestion and reduce symptoms.
8. **Gentle Core Exercises:** Modified planks, bridges, and pelvic tilts can help strengthen the core without putting excessive pressure on the stomach.

9. **Tai Chi:** This slow, flowing exercise can help reduce stress and improve digestion.

10. **Breathing Exercises:** Deep breathing exercises, like diaphragmatic breathing, can help relax the body and reduce symptoms.

Remember to consult with a healthcare provider before starting any new exercise program, especially if you have any underlying health conditions. They can help you develop a personalized exercise plan that suits your needs and health status.

Chapter Five

Managing GERD

Managing GERD requires a combination of lifestyle changes, dietary modifications, and if necessary, medication or surgery.
- Maintain a healthy weight
- Avoid tight clothing
- Quit smoking
- Limit alcohol and caffeine
- Avoid lying down after eating
- Raise the head of your bed

Dietary Modifications:
- Avoid trigger foods (citrus, tomatoes, chocolate, spicy foods)
- Eat smaller, more frequent meals
- Choose low-fat, low-acidity foods
- Avoid carbonated drinks
- Limit processed foods

It's essential to work with a healthcare provider to develop a personalized plan for managing GERD. With appropriate treatment and lifestyle changes, it's possible to alleviate symptoms and improve quality of life.

Managing GERD With Other Health Conditions

Asthma:
1. **Dietary changes:**
   - Avoid trigger foods that can worsen both GERD and asthma
   - Increase omega-3 fatty acid intake, which can help reduce inflammation
2. **Lifestyle modifications:**
   - Maintain a healthy weight, as excess weight can worsen both conditions
   - Avoid lying down after eating or at night, to reduce acid reflux and asthma symptoms
3. **Medication management:**
   - Use inhalers as prescribed for asthma, and antacids or acid reducers for GERD
   - Consider medications that treat both conditions, like montelukast (Singulair)
4. **Breathing exercises:**
   - Practice diaphragmatic breathing to reduce stress and improve lung function
5. **Monitoring and tracking:**
   - Keep a symptom journal to track GERD and asthma symptoms, and adjust treatment plans accordingly
6. **Stress management:**
   - Stress can exacerbate both conditions; engage in stress-reducing activities like yoga or meditation
7. **Consult a specialist:**

- Work with a gastroenterologist and a pulmonologist to develop a comprehensive treatment plan

Some important notes:
- GERD can trigger asthma symptoms, so managing acid reflux is crucial
- Asthma medications can relax the lower esophageal sphincter, worsening GERD symptoms
- Treating both conditions simultaneously can improve overall health and quality of life

Chronic Cough:
1. **Dietary changes:**
   - Avoid trigger foods that can worsen GERD and cough
   - Increase fiber and water intake to thin out mucus
2. **Lifestyle modifications:**
   - Elevate the head of the bed to reduce acid reflux and coughing at night
   - Avoid lying down after eating or drinking
   - Quit smoking and avoid secondhand smoke
3. **Medication management:**
   - Use antacids or acid reducers for GERD
   - Consider cough suppressants or expectorants for chronic cough
   - Inhalers like ipratropium bromide (Atrovent) can help with both GERD and chronic cough
4. **Throat clearing and coughing** techniques:
   - Practice gentle throat clearing and coughing to reduce irritation

5. **Breathing exercises:**
   - Diaphragmatic breathing can help reduce
stress and improve lung function
6. Stress management:
   - Stress can exacerbate both conditions; engage
in stress-reducing activities like yoga or meditation
7. **Consult a specialist:**
   - Work with a gastroenterologist and a
pulmonologist to develop a comprehensive
treatment plan

Some important notes:
- GERD can trigger a chronic cough, as stomach
acid flows up into the esophagus and irritates the
lining, triggering a cough reflex
- A chronic cough can also worsen GERD
symptoms, as coughing can relax the lower
esophageal sphincter and allow acid to flow back
up into the esophagus
- Managing both conditions simultaneously can
improve overall health and quality of life

Obesity:
1. **Weight loss:**
   - Gradual weight loss can help alleviate GERD
symptoms
   - Aim for a healthy BMI (body mass index)
2. **Dietary changes:**
   - Eat smaller, more frequent meals
   - Avoid fatty, spicy, or acidic foods
   - Choose low-fat, low-acid foods like fruits,
vegetables, and whole grains

3. **Lifestyle modifications:**
   - Exercise regularly, like walking or yoga
   - Avoid tight clothing that can worsen symptoms
   - Elevate the head of the bed to reduce acid reflux
4. **Medication management:**
   - Use antacids or acid reducers as prescribed
   - Consider medications that help with weight loss, like orlistat (Alli)
5. **Monitoring and tracking:**
   - Keep a food diary to track eating habits and symptoms
   - Monitor weight loss progress and adjust diet and exercise plans accordingly
6. **Stress management:**
   - Stress can exacerbate both conditions; engage in stress-reducing activities like meditation or deep breathing
7. **Consult a specialist:**
   - Work with a gastroenterologist and a registered dietitian to develop a personalized plan

Some important notes:
- Obesity can worsen GERD symptoms, so weight loss is crucial
- GERD symptoms can improve with weight loss, even without medication
- Lifestyle changes can benefit both conditions, improving overall health

Diabetics:
1. **Dietary changes:**

- Follow a diabetes-friendly diet that is low in sugar, salt, and saturated fats
- Choose foods that are gentle on the stomach, like whole grains, fruits, and vegetables
- Avoid trigger foods that can worsen GERD symptoms

2. **Blood sugar control:**
- Monitor blood sugar levels regularly
- Maintain tight blood sugar control to reduce inflammation and alleviate GERD symptoms

3. **Medication management:**
- Use antacids or acid reducers as prescribed
- Consider medications that help manage blood sugar levels, like metformin (Glucophage)

4. **Lifestyle modifications:**
- Exercise regularly, like walking or yoga
- Maintain a healthy weight to reduce pressure on the stomach
- Avoid lying down after eating or drinking

5. **Monitoring and tracking:**
- Keep a food diary to track eating habits and symptoms
- Monitor blood sugar levels and adjust diet and exercise plans accordingly

6. **Stress management:**
- Stress can exacerbate both conditions; engage in stress-reducing activities like meditation or deep breathing

7. **Consult a specialist:**
- Work with a gastroenterologist, endocrinologist, and registered dietitian to develop a personalized plan

Some important notes:
- Diabetes can increase the risk of developing GERD
- GERD symptoms can worsen blood sugar control
- Managing both conditions simultaneously can improve overall health and quality of life

Osteoporosis:
1. **Dietary changes:**
   - Follow a diet rich in calcium and vitamin D for osteoporosis
   - Choose foods that are gentle on the stomach, like whole grains, fruits, and vegetables
   - Avoid trigger foods that can worsen GERD symptoms
2. **Bone health:**
   - Maintain adequate calcium and vitamin D levels
   - Consider bone density testing and osteoporosis medications if necessary
3. **Medication management:**
   - Use antacids or acid reducers that are safe for osteoporosis treatment
   - Avoid long-term use of proton pump inhibitors (PPIs), which can interfere with calcium absorption
4. **Lifestyle modifications:**
   - Exercise regularly, like walking or yoga, to improve bone density
   - Avoid heavy lifting or bending, which can worsen GERD symptoms
   - Maintain a healthy weight to reduce pressure on the stomach and bones

5. **Monitoring and tracking:**
   - Keep a food diary to track eating habits and symptoms
   - Monitor bone density and adjust diet and exercise plans accordingly
6. **Stress management:**
   - Stress can exacerbate both conditions; engage in stress-reducing activities like meditation or deep breathing
7. **Consult a specialist:**
   - Work with a gastroenterologist, endocrinologist, and registered dietitian to develop a personalized plan

Some important notes:
- Osteoporosis medications like alendronate (Fosamax) can worsen GERD symptoms
- GERD symptoms can lead to poor nutrition, which can worsen osteoporosis
- Managing both conditions simultaneously can improve overall health and quality of life

Fibromyalgia:
1. **Dietary changes:**
   - Follow a gentle, easy-to-digest diet that avoids trigger foods
   - Choose foods rich in omega-3 fatty acids, like fish and flaxseeds, to reduce inflammation
2. **Stress management:**
   - Stress can exacerbate both conditions; engage in stress-reducing activities like meditation, yoga, or deep breathing

3. **Sleep hygiene:**
   - Establish a consistent sleep schedule to manage fatigue and pain
   - Avoid lying down after eating or drinking
4. **Pain management:**
   - Work with your healthcare provider to manage fibromyalgia pain
   - Avoid medications that can irritate the stomach, like NSAIDs
5. **Lifestyle modifications:**
   - Exercise regularly, like walking or swimming, to reduce pain and improve digestion
   - Practice relaxation techniques, like progressive muscle relaxation or visualization
6. **Monitoring and tracking:**
   - Keep a food diary to track eating habits and symptoms
   - Monitor pain levels and adjust diet and exercise plans accordingly
7. **Consult a specialist:**
   - Work with a gastroenterologist, rheumatologist, and registered dietitian to develop a personalized plan

Some important notes:
- Fibromyalgia can increase sensitivity to acid reflux and worsen GERD symptoms
- GERD symptoms can worsen fibromyalgia pain and fatigue
- Managing both conditions simultaneously can improve overall health and quality of life

Irritable Bowel Syndrome (IBS)
1. **Dietary changes:**
   - Follow a low-FODMAP diet to manage IBS symptoms
   - Avoid trigger foods that can worsen GERD symptoms
   - Choose foods that are gentle on the stomach, like bananas, rice, applesauce, and toast (BRAT diet)
2. **Gut health:**
   - Maintain a healthy gut microbiome through probiotics or prebiotics
   - Consider a low-acid, high-fiber diet to promote gut health
3. **Stress management:**
   - Stress can exacerbate both conditions; engage in stress-reducing activities like meditation, yoga, or deep breathing
4. **Bowel habits:**
   - Establish a regular bowel routine to manage IBS symptoms
   - Avoid straining during bowel movements, which can worsen GERD symptoms
5. **Lifestyle modifications:**
   - Exercise regularly, like walking or yoga, to reduce stress and improve digestion
   - Avoid tight clothing that can worsen GERD symptoms
6. **Monitoring and tracking:**
   - Keep a food diary to track eating habits and symptoms

- Monitor bowel movements and adjust diet and exercise plans accordingly

7. **Consult a specialist:**

   - Work with a gastroenterologist and registered dietitian to develop a personalized plan

Some important notes:
- IBS can increase sensitivity to acid reflux and worsen GERD symptoms
- GERD symptoms can worsen IBS symptoms, creating a cycle of discomfort
- Managing both conditions simultaneously can improve overall health and quality of life

Sleep Apnea:

1. **Lifestyle modifications:**

   - Lose weight, if overweight or obese, to reduce symptoms of both conditions
   - Avoid alcohol, smoking, and sedatives, which can worsen both GERD and sleep apnea
   - Sleep on your side or elevate the head of your bed to reduce acid reflux

2. **Dietary changes:**

   - Avoid heavy meals close to bedtime
   - Choose foods that are easy to digest and low in acid, like fruits, vegetables, and whole grains

3. **Sleep hygiene:**

   - Establish a consistent sleep schedule and create a relaxing sleep environment
   - Avoid screens and stimulating activities before bedtime

4. **Breathing exercises:**

- Practice nasal breathing exercises to improve nasal passages and reduce snoring

5. **CPAP therapy:**
- Use continuous positive airway pressure (CPAP) therapy as prescribed for sleep apnea
- Consider using a CPAP machine with a humidifier to reduce acid reflux

6. **Medication management:**
- Use antacids or acid reducers as prescribed for GERD
- Consider medications that help manage sleep apnea, like modafinil (Provigil)

7. **Consult a specialist:**
- Work with a gastroenterologist, pulmonologist, and sleep specialist to develop a personalized plan

Some important notes:
- Sleep apnea can increase the risk of developing GERD
- GERD symptoms can worsen sleep apnea, creating a cycle of discomfort
- Managing both conditions simultaneously can improve overall health and quality of life

During Pregnancy:

1. **Dietary changes:**
- Eat smaller, frequent meals
- Avoid spicy, fatty, or acidic foods
- Choose soft, easy-to-digest foods like bananas, rice, applesauce, and toast (BRAT diet)

2. **Lifestyle modifications:**
- Avoid lying down after eating or drinking

- Elevate the head of your bed by 6-8 inches
- Avoid tight clothing that can worsen symptoms

3. **Natural remedies:**
- Ginger: try ginger tea, ginger ale, or ginger candies
- Acupuncture: may help alleviate symptoms

4. **Medication management:**
- Antacids like Tums, Rolaids, or Mylanta are generally safe during pregnancy
- Acid reducers like Zantac or Pepcid may be prescribed by your doctor

5. **Monitoring and tracking:**
- Keep a food diary to track eating habits and symptoms
- Monitor your baby's growth and development

6. **Consult a specialist:**
- Work with your obstetrician and a gastroenterologist to develop a personalized plan

Some important notes:
- Hormonal changes during pregnancy can relax the lower esophageal sphincter, worsening GERD symptoms
- GERD symptoms can worsen as the pregnancy progresses and the uterus expands
- Managing GERD during pregnancy can help alleviate symptoms and prevent complications

Natural Remedies And Alternative Therapies

1. **Ginger:** Has natural anti-inflammatory properties that may help reduce inflammation and alleviate symptoms.
2. **Aloe vera juice:** May help soothe the esophagus and reduce inflammation.
3. **Licorice root:** Has anti-inflammatory properties that may help reduce inflammation and alleviate symptoms.
4. **Slippery elm:** May help soothe and protect the mucous membranes in the esophagus.
5. **Acupuncture:** May help reduce symptoms by improving digestion and reducing stress.
6. **Chiropractic care:** May help improve digestion and reduce stress by aligning the spine.
7. **Massage therapy:** May help reduce stress and improve digestion.
8. **Yoga and meditation:** May help reduce stress and improve digestion.
9. **Probiotics:** May help maintain a healthy gut microbiome and improve digestion.
10. **Digestive enzymes:** May help improve digestion and reduce symptoms.

When To seek Medical Attention

1. Severe chest pain or difficulty breathing
2. Vomiting blood or black tarry stools
3. Difficulty swallowing or painful swallowing

4. Heartburn that worsens at night or interferes with daily activities
5. GERD symptoms that don't improve with lifestyle changes or medication
6. Unintentional weight loss
7. Hoarseness or wheezing
8. Coughing or choking on food
9. Feeling like food is stuck in your throat
10. Severe abdominal pain or tenderness

Additionally,if you have a history of GERD and experience any of the following, seek medical attention:
1. Increased frequency or severity of symptoms
2. Difficulty managing symptoms with usual medications
3. New or worsening symptoms
4. Symptoms that interfere with daily activities or sleep

Remember, if you're unsure about your symptoms or concerns, it's always best to consult with a healthcare professional for proper evaluation and guidance.

Conclusion

Gastroesophageal reflux disease (GERD) is a chronic condition that affects millions of people worldwide, causing discomfort, pain, and disruption to daily life. However, with the right combination of lifestyle changes, dietary modifications, and medical treatment, it is possible to manage symptoms, prevent complications, and improve quality of life.

By understanding the causes, symptoms, and treatment options for GERD, individuals can take control of their health and make informed decisions about their care. Whether through medication, surgery, or natural remedies, there are many effective ways to alleviate symptoms and prevent long-term damage to the esophagus.

Remember, if you're experiencing symptoms of GERD, don't hesitate to speak with your healthcare provider. With the right treatment and lifestyle changes, you can find relief from this common condition and enjoy a healthier, happier life. Take control of your health and don't let GERD hold you back.

Encouragement To Take Control Of GERD Management

You have the power to take control of your GERD management. By making small changes to your daily habits and working with your healthcare provider, you can alleviate symptoms, prevent complications, and improve your overall quality of life.

Remember, managing GERD is a journey, and it's okay to take it one step at a time. Start with small changes, like adjusting your diet or exercise routine, and build from there.

Don't let GERD hold you back from enjoying life's moments. Take control of your health and well-being, and know that you're capable of managing your symptoms and living a healthy, happy life.

You got this.

Appendix

Grocery List

Fruits:
- Bananas
- Melons (cantaloupe, honeydew, watermelon)
- Berries (strawberries, blueberries, raspberries)
- Apples
- Pears
- Peaches
- Apricots
- Plums
- Grapes

Vegetables:
- Leafy greens (spinach, kale, collard greens)
- Broccoli
- Cauliflower
- Carrots
- Green beans
- Sweet potatoes
- Peas
- Cucumbers
- Bell peppers

Proteins:
- Lean beef
- Chicken
- Turkey
- Fish (cod, salmon, tilapia)

- Tofu
- Legumes (lentils, chickpeas, black beans)

Grains:
- Whole wheat bread
- Brown rice
- Quinoa
- Oatmeal
- Whole-grain pasta
- Whole-grain cereals

Dairy:
- Low-fat milk
- Low-fat yogurt
- Low-fat cheese
- Almond milk
- Soy milk

Healthy Fats:
- Avocado
- Nuts (almonds, walnuts, pecans)
- Seeds (chia, flax, sunflower)
- Olive oil

Beverages
-Herbal tea
- Low-acidity juice (apple, grape)
- Almond milk
- Soy milk
-Water
-fats

Condiments:
- Salt
- Pepper
- Herbs (basil, oregano, thyme)
- Spices (cumin, coriander, ginger)
- Low-acidic salad dressings

2 Weeks Meal Plan

Day 1:
- Breakfast: Oatmeal with sliced banana, almond butter, and a splash of low-fat milk
- Lunch: Grilled chicken breast with roasted vegetables (such as zucchini, bell peppers, and onions) and quinoa
- Snack: Apple slices with a tablespoon of almond butter
- Dinner: Baked salmon with sweet potato and green beans

Day 2:
- Breakfast: Greek yogurt with mixed berries and whole-grain granola
- Lunch: Turkey and avocado wrap with mixed greens and a whole-grain tortilla
- Snack: Cottage cheese with sliced cucumber
- Dinner: Grilled turkey burger on a whole-grain bun with roasted carrots and a side salad

Day 3:
- Breakfast: Smoothie bowl with almond milk, spinach, banana, and whole-grain granola
- Snack: Rice cakes with almond butter and banana slices
- Lunch: Chicken Caesar salad with whole-grain croutons and a light Caesar dressing
- Dinner: Slow-cooked lentil soup with whole-grain bread

Day 4:
- Breakfast: Scrambled eggs with whole-grain toast and sautéed spinach
- Lunch: Grilled chicken breast with mixed greens and a balsamic vinaigrette dressing
- Snack: Apple slices with a tablespoon of peanut butter
- Dinner: Baked cod with roasted asparagus and brown rice

Day 5:
- Breakfast: Avocado toast on whole-grain bread with scrambled eggs
- Lunch: Turkey and cheese sandwich on whole-grain bread with a side salad
- Snack: Rice crackers with almond butter and banana slices
- Dinner: Grilled shrimp with quinoa and steamed broccoli

Day 6:
- Breakfast: Whole-grain waffles with fresh berries and yogurt
- Lunch: Chicken and vegetable stir-fry with brown rice
- Snack: Cottage cheese with sliced cucumber
- Dinner: Baked chicken breast with roasted Brussels sprouts and sweet potato

Day 7:
- Breakfast: Whole-grain cereal with almond milk and sliced banana

- Snack: Hard-boiled egg and a small serving of whole-grain crackers
- Lunch: Grilled chicken wrap with mixed greens and whole-grain tortilla
- Snack: Apple slices with a tablespoon of almond butter
- Dinner: Slow-cooked beef stew with whole-grain bread

Day 8:
- Breakfast: Omelette with vegetables (such as bell peppers, onions, and mushrooms) and whole-grain toast
- Snack: Greek yogurt with mixed berries and a sprinkle of granola
- Lunch: Grilled chicken breast with roasted vegetables and quinoa
- Dinner: Baked salmon with sweet potato and green beans

Day 9:
- Breakfast: Whole-grain English muffin with scrambled eggs and avocado
- Snack: Protein smoothie with almond milk, banana, and spinach
- Lunch: Turkey and cheese sandwich on whole-grain bread with a side salad
- Dinner: Grilled shrimp with quinoa and steamed asparagus

Day 10:
- Breakfast: Whole-grain pancakes with fresh berries and yogurt
- Lunch: Chicken Caesar salad with whole-grain croutons and a light Caesar dressing
- Snack: Apple slices with a tablespoon of peanut butter
- Dinner: Slow-cooked lentil soup with whole-grain bread

Day 11:
- Breakfast: Avocado toast on whole-grain bread with scrambled eggs
- Snack: Greek yogurt with mixed berries and a sprinkle of granola
- Lunch: Grilled chicken breast with mixed greens and a balsamic vinaigrette dressing
- Dinner: Baked cod with roasted Brussels sprouts and brown rice

Day 12:
- Breakfast: Whole-grain waffles with fresh berries and yogurt
- Lunch: Turkey and avocado wrap with mixed greens and whole-grain tortilla
- Snack: Rice crackers with almond butter and banana slices
- Dinner: Grilled chicken breast with roasted carrots and sweet potato

Day 13:
- Breakfast: Oatmeal with sliced banana, almond butter, and a splash of low-fat milk
- Lunch: Grilled chicken Caesar salad with whole-grain croutons and a light Caesar dressing
- Snack: Apple slices with a tablespoon of almond butter
- Dinner: Slow-cooked beef stew with whole-grain bread

Day 14:
- Breakfast: Whole-grain cereal with almond milk and sliced banana
- Lunch: Grilled chicken wrap with mixed greens and whole-grain tortilla
- Snack: Carrot sticks with hummus
- Dinner: Baked salmon with roasted asparagus and quinoa

Remember to stay hydrated by drinking plenty of water throughout the day. Avoid trigger foods and adjust the portion sizes based on your individual needs.

Meal Plan Template

Monday
- Breakfast:

____

____

- Lunch:

____

____

- Dinner:

____

____

Remark:

____

____

Tuesday
- Breakfast:

____

____

- Lunch:

____

____

- Dinner:

____

____

Remark:

____

____

Wednesday

- Breakfast:

____

____

- Lunch:

____

____

- Dinner:

____

____

Remark:

____

____

Thursday
- Breakfast:

____

____

- Lunch:

____

____

- Dinner:

____

____

Remark:

____

____

Friday
- Breakfast:

____

____

- Lunch:
____
____
- Dinner:
____
____
Remark:
____
____

Saturday
- Breakfast:
____
____
- Lunch:
____
____
- Dinner:
____
____
Remark:
____
____

Sunday
- Breakfast:
____
____
- Lunch:
____
____

- Dinner:

____

Remark:

____

____

Grocery List

Produce:

____

____

____

____

____

____

Proteins:

____

____

____

____

____

____

Grains:

____

____

____
____
____
____

Dairy:

____
____
____
____
____

Pantry:

____
____
____
____
____

You can fill in the meal plan template with your desired meals and then use the grocery list section to write down the ingredients you need to buy. You can also adjust the categories in the grocery list section based on your personal needs.